How to Become a Healthier, Prettier You

Books by Mary Ellen

MARY ELLEN'S BEST OF HELPFUL HINTS
MARY ELLEN'S BEST OF HELPFUL KITCHEN HINTS
MARY ELLEN'S BEST OF HELPFUL HINTS BOOK II
MARY ELLEN'S HELP YOURSELF DIET PLAN
MARY ELLEN'S 1,000 NEW HELPFUL HINTS

How to Become a Healthier, Prettier You

THE LATEST ON NUTRITION, DIET, EXERCISE, AND BEAUTY

By Mary Ellen Pinkham

Illustrations by Lynn Johnston

DOUBLEDAY & COMPANY, INC.
GARDEN CITY, NEW YORK
1984

The hints in this book are intended to suggest possible solutions only. The author and publisher cannot guarantee absolute success. For best and safest results, we recommend following these hints with care.

ISBN 0-385-19359-9

PRINTED IN THE UNITED STATES OF AMERICA
FIRST EDITION

Library of Congress Cataloging in Publication Data

Pinkham, Mary Ellen.
How to become a healthier, prettier you.

Includes index.
1. Health. 2. Women—Health and hygiene. 3. Beauty, Personal. I. Title. II. Title: How to become a healthier, prettier you.
RA776.P64 1984 613'.04244 84-8145

Introduction

Some people like to collect things, I like to collect hints. For one thing, they don't have to be dusted.

Also, unlike many collectibles, good hints can be put to use. I have gathered and shared some terrific ones in my books.

Most of my hints related to things, and as a result everything in my life was in pretty good shape. Everything, that is, except me. I knew more about removing stains than removing stress. I paid more attention to maintaining my car's body than my own.

Until a couple of years ago. That's when I put down my cake fork, put on my walking shoes, and lost seventy pounds. As I got trimmer and healthier, I became interested in getting even more trim, more fit, and more healthy. So, naturally, I began looking for hints on the subject.

This book is a collection of those hints. Some are just interesting to think about: Did you know that chocolate and romance have the same effects on your body? Some contradict ideas I always had: It's not true that you should feed a cold and starve a fever. Some made me more cautious: Hot dogs and honey can be dangerous for kids. And some were unexpectedly good news: Cheaper meat is better for dieters. All of them helped to make my life better in some way.

While none of the hints in this collection may change your life overnight, there are many that may help you get a better start tomorrow morning, either by solving your insomnia problem, suggesting a better method to brush your teeth, or recommending a way to keep your orange juice packed with vitamins. I truly believe that among them you'll find many that will make a difference.

So, start reading. Here's to your health!

Mary Ellen

Contents

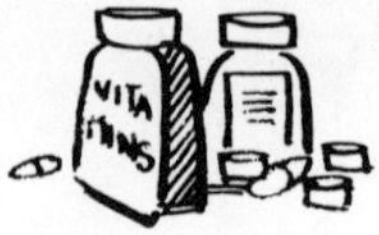

Chapter 1

Here's to Eating Right NUTRITION

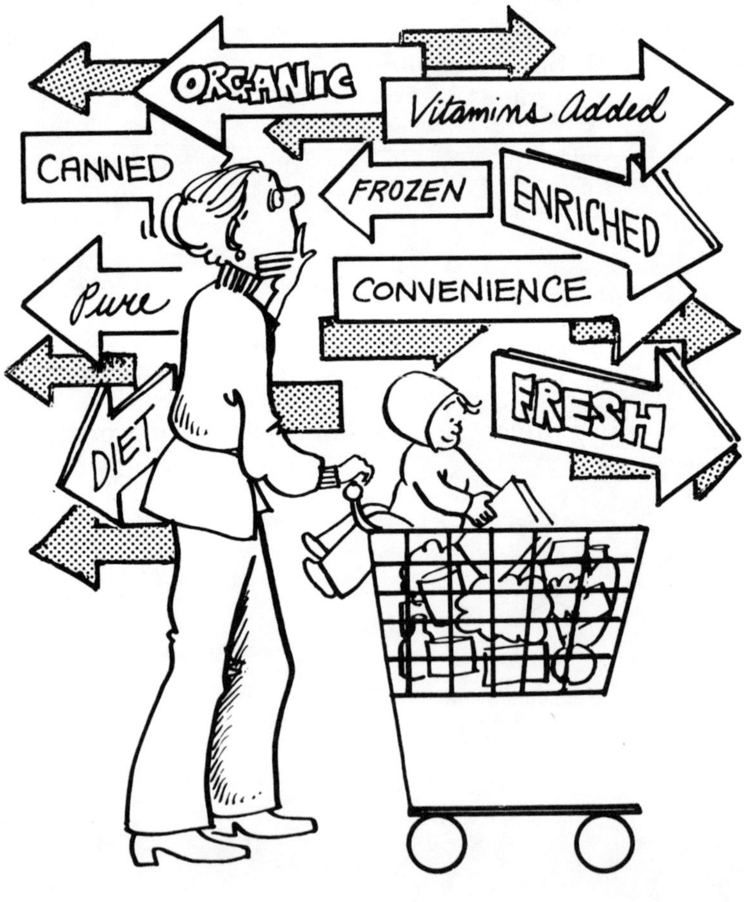

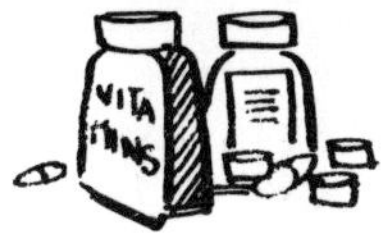

The Typical American Diet

No wonder you're full!

- If you're an average American, last year you ate 150 pounds of red meat, 48 pounds of chicken, 35 pounds of eggs (about 260 of them), 10 pounds of turkey, 13 pounds of fish, 290 pounds of milk and cream, 12 pounds of margarine, 80 pounds of fresh fruit, 125 pounds of potatoes, 95 pounds of other fresh vegetables, 112 pounds of wheat flour, 7 pounds of coffee, and 93 pounds of refined sugar.

Eating less . . . and more

- You're probably eating fewer calories and more nutrients than you did fifteen years ago, but also eating more processed and "fast" foods that are less nutritious and have more additives and preservatives.

Most popular foods

- Milk, meat, and potatoes are what you eat most of, followed by sugar, canned vegetables, fresh fruit other than citrus, pork, chicken, eggs, fresh citrus fruit.

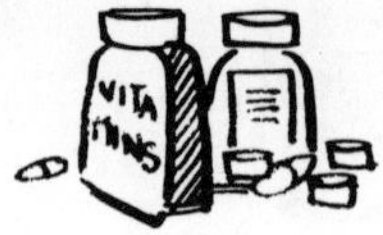

Nutrition Facts and Myths

Did you know . . .

- The best time to take vitamins is after a meal, not before. It's the interaction with food in your stomach that makes them effective.

Too much of a good thing

- Don't waste money buying food with vitamins and minerals added if you've already got enough in your diet. The body uses only what it needs, so the extra is useless and, in rare cases, may actually be toxic.
- Vitamins A and D and the minerals copper and zinc can be poisonous in excess. Ask your doctor for a recommended dosage.
- Excesses of vitamin C, which usually prevents scurvy, can actually *cause* the disease. If you take enormous dosages, then cut back suddenly, you may suffer "rebound scurvy." If you're on more than 1,000 to 2,000 mg. daily, cut back—but do it slowly.

Natural or chemical?

- "Natural" and man-made vitamins are equally effective, no matter what claims the health faddists make.

Are your vitamins potent?

- Vitamins can lose up to half their strength if they're old or improperly stored.
- Your vitamins are likely to be fresher if you buy them from a busy store where the turnover is fast.

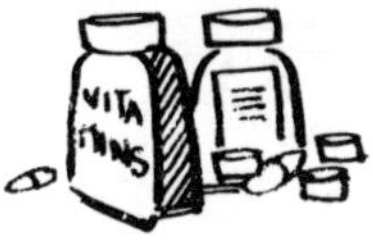

- Check the expiration date on vitamins and avoid those that do not have it in print.
- Buy in small quantities.
- At home, store the vitamins out of sunlight and away from moisture. If you keep them tightly capped, in a cool, dry closet, they'll keep for up to two years.

Your calcium intake

- It's very likely that you aren't getting enough calcium. Women need 1,000 to 1,500 mg. of calcium a day, the equivalent of three glasses of milk. Besides milk, other good sources are milk products such as yogurt or cheese, broccoli, sardines, lentils.
- People at one point were concerned that an essential element in chocolate—oxalic acid—prevented calcium in milk from being absorbed. However, this has recently been proved false.
- You may not be getting enough calcium if you drink lots of cola, eat more than 6 oz. of meat a day, or eat a lot of fats, because all these prevent the absorption of calcium.

Your potassium needs

- Diuretics may increase your need for potassium.
- You may also need more potassium in the summer, when you perspire more and are likely to eat less.
- Foods richest in potassium are bananas, cooked beet greens, baked sweet or white potatoes, baked winter squash, broccoli, cooked chard, canned tomato sauce and paste and lima beans.
- Potassium-rich foods are exceptionally low in sodium.

Chocolate lovers

- When you're in love your brain releases a special chemical

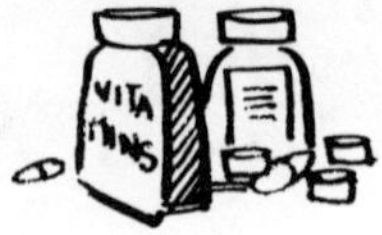

into your system—a chemical also found in chocolate. That's why, when you're not getting real kisses, your body may crave chocolate ones.

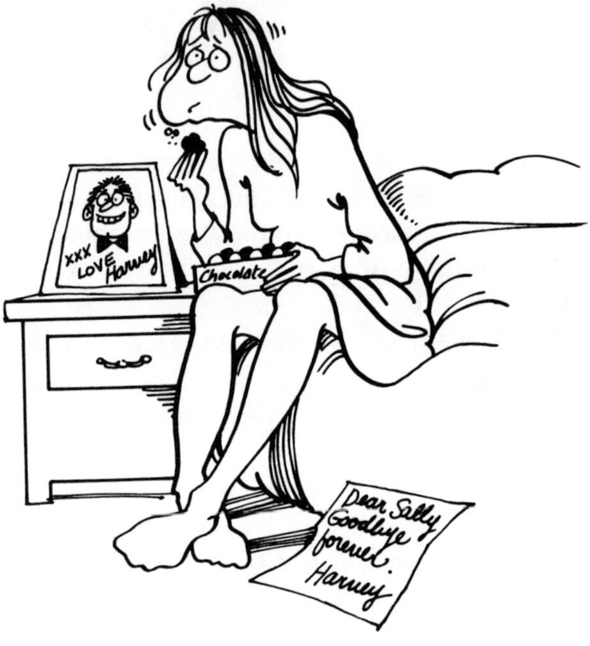

Eating the blues away

- Turkey, chicken, bananas, cheese, pineapple, and yogurt may relieve depression in combination with foods rich in B vitamins like whole grains, green vegetables, organ meats, brown rice. So a turkey sandwich on whole wheat bread may give you a boost.
- But if you're feeling low, avoid lobster and egg yolks: the cholesterol brings you down.

B vitamins—natural pep-up

- Brewer's yeast is the best source of all the B vitamins ex-

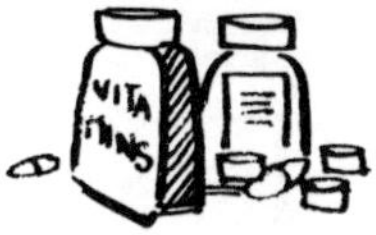

cept B_{12} (which is generally added to it). Disguise the icky taste by adding it to orange juice.

- Both coffee and tea destroy vitamin B_1.
- Lightly toasted bread retains more of the B vitamins than dark toast.

Three squares a day

- Breakfast is not the most important meal nutritionally, as you've always been told. This idea was popularized by (no surprise!) the Cereal Institute. However, it is helpful (especially for dieters) to eat something to start the day: it gets your metabolism going.
- You won't get fatter by eating only one big meal a day. But your body will seesaw between high cholesterol and low blood sugar.

Healthier substitutes

- Good substitutes for salt-loaded, artificially flavored chips are the salt-free kind with no artificial preservatives.
- Or try the new carrot chips if your kids want a snack.
- Try peanut butter made only of freshly ground peanuts with no added sugar or salt.
- Try cookie sandwiches made with graham crackers spread with farmer's or low-fat cream cheese and sliced berries instead of jam.

The gassiest foods

- Along with baked beans, they include milk, milk products, onions, celery, carrots, raisins, bananas, apricots, prune juice, pretzels, bagels, wheat germ and brussels sprouts.
- Most people will find beans less gas-producing if they've been soaked in water for several hours. Though soaking

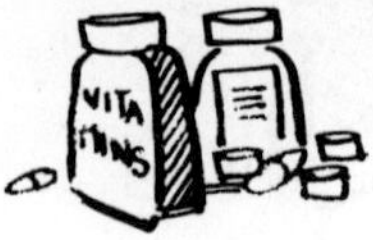

removes some nutrients, it also removes most of the undigestible sugars. Before cooking beans, discard the water they've been soaking in and replace with fresh water.

- Mildly gassy foods include potatoes, eggplants, citrus fruits, apples, bread, and pastry.
- Stomach upset caused by onions, lettuce, or cabbage isn't due to gas but to an irritation of the stomach lining.

The Smart Shopper

If the label doesn't tell you enough

- If you need additional nutritional information about a product—number of calories, amount of salt, etc.—write to the company's consumer affairs division. The address should be on the label.

Buying "health food" at the supermarket

- Fresh foods, grains, and low-salt and low-sugar products are available at most supermarkets, often at prices lower than in the health food stores. Start looking for products new to you that have these advantages.

Is "natural" always better?

- "Natural" potato chips contain exactly the same ingredients as potato chips without the "natural" label. Right now, "natural" means only that the food contains no synthetic or artificial ingredients or additives. Make sure you're not paying extra for the same thing.

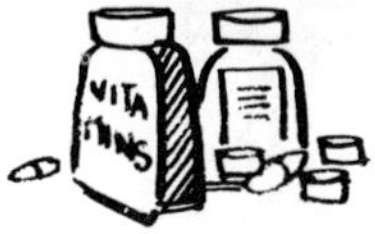

Frankly speaking

- "All meat" frankfurters may contain 10 percent water and 5 percent other ingredients such as spices, flavorings, chemicals. And another 30 percent may be fat.
- And don't think that "all beef" franks include only beef *steak* and other cuts that you would buy at the butcher shop. They include *any* edible parts of a cow.
- Corn syrup is present in most franks.

Nothing's fishy about fish, IF . . .

- You'll know the fish is fresh if it has: clear, bright eyes that protrude slightly; bright red or pink (not dark) gills; a mild, clean smell; a clean intestinal cavity; flesh that springs back when you poke it.

Some like it raw

- If your family likes sushi and steak tartare, make sure the sushi is fresh and the beef is prime and chopped as freshly as possible. Otherwise you may have problems with worms or bacteria.

For freshest chicken

- Properly refrigerated, chicken will stay fresh in the supermarket for at least seven days, so check the date on the package. If you're in an area where packages aren't dated, choose chicken that looks moist and blemish-free and is a light, milky color. Pale birds may be anemic or otherwise unhealthy. A very yellow chicken is either too fatty or, because people have been under the impression that yellow chicken is better, has been fed a diet of marigold seeds. (I prefer my marigold seeds in the garden.)

For the freshest eggs

- Always buy from a refrigerated case. At room tempera-

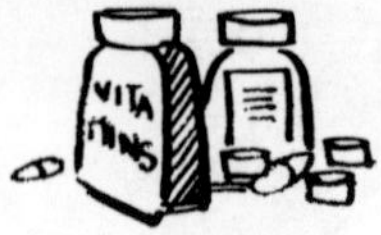

ture an egg loses more quality in one day than it will during a week of refrigeration.

How large is "extra-large"?

- Eggs called extra-large weigh 27 to 30 ounces per dozen. Large weigh 24 to 27 ounces per dozen; medium weigh 21 to 24; and small weigh in at 18 to 21 ounces per dozen. (If only panty-hose sizes were as easy to figure out!)

Brown eggs vs. white

- Brown eggs are not more nutritious than white. The only difference is in the breed of the chicken that lays it.

Fresh vs. frozen

- Frozen fruits or vegetables, often cheaper, may also be more nutritious than fresh. If a fruit or vegetable is picked and then flash-frozen almost immediately, it probably has lost less vitamins A, B, or C than if it's spent a long time in shipment and on your grocer's shelf. Food is *guaranteed* fresh only if you pick it yourself.
- Frozen orange juice has 95 percent or more of the vitamin C of freshly squeezed. One-half cup of fresh juice has 62 mg.; one-half cup of frozen has 60; carton juices have only half of that. (The recommended daily allowance is 60 mg.)

At the fruit and vegetable stand

- These fruits can be bought unripe and will ripen uncovered at home: avocados, bananas, honeydew melons, mangoes, papayas, persimmons.
- Apricots, nectarines, peaches, pears, and plums may be ripened at home in a loosely covered paper bag.
- But these don't get riper, so buy them ready to eat: apples, berries, grapes, grapefruit, pineapples, pomegranates, and rhubarb.

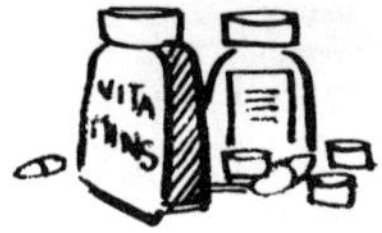

- Always choose oranges, grapefruit, and lemons that are heavy for their size.
- Oranges that have developed green areas are not unripe. They are "regreened"—but they're ready to eat.
- Pass up light-colored salad greens for darker ones and you'll be getting more nutrition for your dollar. For example, use kale or spinach instead of iceberg lettuce.
- If your family eats only "token" vegetables like corn, green beans, and iceberg lettuce, they probably aren't getting enough vitamin C or A.
- The most nutritious fruits and vegetables are the dark green vegetables, green peppers and tomatoes, citrus fruits and melons.

Preventive "medicine"

- Harvard researchers are doing a five-year study to see whether dark green and yellow vegetables (rich in beta-carotene) can prevent certain types of cancer. No matter what the outcome, you should buy and serve daily one or more of those foods, such as spinach, carrots, cantaloupes, beet greens, broccoli, butternut squash.

Go coco-nuts

- Fresh coconuts keep for two months and taste better than the packaged, shredded stuff. To test, shake the coconut. If you can hear the liquid, it's fresh.
- And you don't need to drop it off a ten-story building to get at the milk and meat. Use an ice pick or screwdriver to punch out the three eyes, then drain.
- To get at the meat, bake the coconut in preheated 325-degree oven for 15 minutes and crack it with a hammer. Remove meat, peel away dark skin, and shred in a food processor.
- If you grate the meat by hand, use a medium grater.

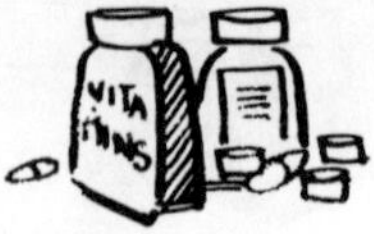

Berry good selections

- Choose smaller blueberries and strawberries. They're sweeter than the monster ones. (You knew good things came in small packages.)
- Also, choose berries with caps. If they're gone, the berries may be too ripe.
- Wash strawberries with caps on and *then* hull, to preserve juices.

Ripening on the vine

- If the stem is still attached or the scar is jagged, a melon was taken from the vine too early. If the cantaloupe is ripe, the stem scar will be smooth.

Do you need "fortified" breakfast cereals?

- "Fortified" cereals provide 100 percent of the RDA (recommended daily allowance) of certain nutrients (and, interestingly, none at all of others). But since you'll probably get a certain amount of these nutrients in your diet anyway, you may be wasting money by paying extra for them in cereal form.

Keeping Food Nutritious

Bacon

- Use it within a week. Maximum recommended refrigerator storage time for bacon and other smoked meats (franks, hams) is seven days.
- The FDA says that slab bacon, tightly wrapped, may be frozen for 1 to 3 months, but the sliced kind shouldn't be frozen at all.

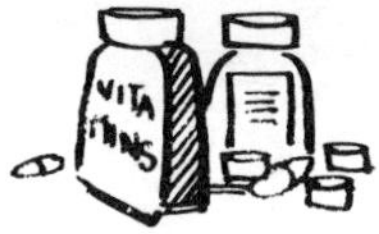

Bananas

- Go ahead and refrigerate them. The skin may turn brown, but the fruit is fine.

Berries and cherries

- They'll last longer if you store them unwashed and uncovered. Leave caps and stems on, too.

Canned goods

- If you store canned goods in a cool place, you'll keep vitamin loss to a minimum. Don't put them over the stove or fridge.
- The FDA says you may keep most food in the can after it's been opened. But remove acidic foods such as pineapple or tomatoes and store in glass or plastic containers. The acid may corrode the can, and juices could take on lead.

Carrots

- Leaves draw moisture away from the vegetable. So cut off the tops before you put the carrots in your crisper.

Dried peas and beans

- Keep in a dark container or they lose vitamins A and B.

Dried fruits

- They'll stay moist if you refrigerate them.

Eggs

- Never wash them before storing. Germs are more likely to penetrate the porous shell.
- Store eggs in their own carton, not in the refrigerator egg shelf, and they'll keep longer. And if you store eggs with the large ends up they'll stay fresher.
- Yolks may be kept in the fridge for up to two days. Pour

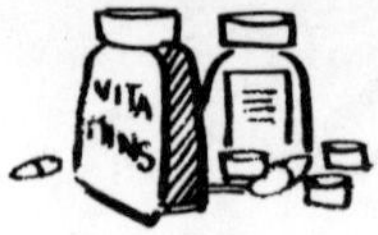

a bit of cold water on top and keep them in a closed container. Pour off the water when you're ready to use the yolks.

- If you're having trouble peeling an egg, you can at least be assured it's fresh. Fresh ones are hardest to peel after boiling.
- A fresh egg covers a small area when it's cracked into a pan, while the yolk remains round and upstanding and the white firm and thick around the yolk. An old, low-quality egg spreads thinly in the pan and the yolk flattens and breaks easily.

Frozen food

- It's best not to refreeze any thawed raw food. But cooked food, such as leftover turkey, that has been *slightly* thawed may be refrozen if it's still below 40 degrees or if ice crystals are present.
- If raw food has thawed, you may cook it and *then* refreeze it.
- Rule of thumb: The thicker the meat, the longer it keeps in the freezer. It's less vulnerable to freezer burn and dehydration.
- Definitely do not refreeze ice cream (because the texture will change), frozen juice (because you lose vitamins), or anything creamed, such as vegetables or meats or cream pies (because of possible contamination).
- Freezing fruits in juices enriched with vitamin C will help prevent browning. (Juice is lower in calories than syrup, too.)
- Thaw food in the fridge, allowing six hours per pound. If you must thaw at room temperature, allow three hours per pound, and cook the food while it's still cool to be sure it hasn't been contaminated.

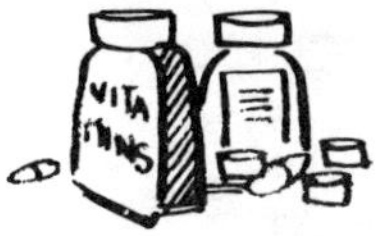

- Don't keep your freezer in a cold room such as an unheated garage. It may not operate properly in the cold, and your food may spoil.
- The USDA suggests these maximum storage times (at 0 degrees) for meats: fresh whole poultry, beef roasts and steaks, 12 months; lamb roasts, lamb chops, chicken parts, 9 months; pork and veal roast, 8 months; turkey pieces, 6 months; pork chops, variety meats, ground and stew meats, 4 months; pork sausages, 3 months.

Fruit
- The more you slice them, the more surface area you expose and the greater the loss of nutrients. Cut-up citrus fruits may lose a quarter of their vitamin C in a day.
- Don't slice or skin until just before serving. But if you must, cover the fruit with lemon and/or orange juice and store in a covered container. That cuts nutrient loss, keeps fruit from turning brown.
- Fruit keeps best if it's unwashed. But when you're ready to use it, wash it thoroughly to remove all traces of chemicals.
- Long storage periods lead to loss of nutrients. Cover fruits and vegetables well once they have been cut.

Grains
- Whole-wheat flour and brown rice will last up to a year in the fridge, only six months at room temperature.

Grapefruit
- Store it in the refrigerator, covered with aluminum foil or waxed paper to prevent it drying out. Plastic rots it.

Honey
- Honey (and syrup) won't get moldy if refrigerated and will

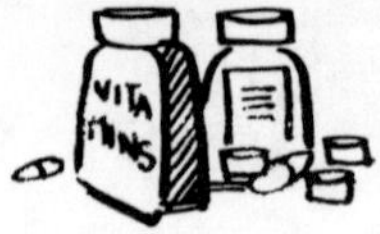

stay fresh up to a year. If they crystallize, just heat the jar in warm water.

Juice

- Store orange juice made from frozen concentrate in a closed container or it will lose up to 15 percent of its vitamin C per day.

Leftovers

- Putting them in the fridge while they're hot may raise your refrigerator's temperature, risking spoilage of other foods. Cool leftovers quickly by placing the covered container in a pan of cold water, then refrigerate.
- Wrap food before refrigerating but after cooling down, as condensation inside the wrapper may cause bacterial growth.

Lettuce

- If you're planning to serve the salad right away, go ahead and chop—it's quicker. But if you plan to store lettuce, tear it: the edges won't darken as quickly.

Mayonnaise salads

- You used to hear that salads with mayonnaise spoil quickly, but recent studies say it's not so. Its acidity (from vinegar and/or lemon) actually prevents or halts harmful bacteria growth.

Meat and poultry

- All meat and poultry should be kept partially dry in the refrigerator to avoid bacterial growth. So remove plastic wrap that clings too tightly to allow drying.
- Before you repack and store it, wipe the meat or poultry dry with a cloth or paper towel.

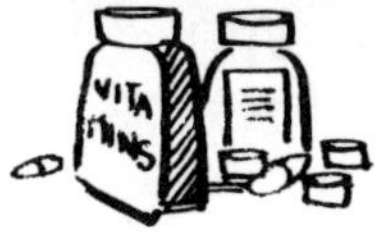

- The USDA has a food safety inspection service (FSIS) to answer any questions about preparation and storage of meat and poultry. Call 202-472-4485 or write FSIS Meat and Poultry Hotline, USDA, Washington, D.C. 20250, including your address and daytime phone number. They may telephone you.

Milk
- Milk shouldn't be stored in the door, but in the coldest part of the refrigerator.
- Vitamins A and B are destroyed by light. So store milk in its carton, not in a glass pitcher.
- UHT (Ultra High Temperature) milk can keep on your shelf and doesn't need refrigeration until it's opened. It's the same nutritionally as regular milk. It may cost a bit more, though.

Non-dairy creamer
- It belongs in the fridge, not on the pantry shelf—especially in hot, humid climates.

Nuts
- Keep in the fridge, where they'll stay fresh for six months, or in the freezer for up to a year.

Oils
- Keep oils in the fridge to keep them fresh. They may get cloudy, but they'll look fine once they're back at room temperature. (Olive oil and sesame oil will keep only 1 to 2 months on the shelf, or 6 to 8 months in the fridge.)

Undated foods
- Use a small date stamp or stick-on label when you put spices, flour, or other items in your own container or when

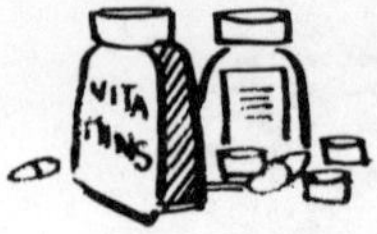

you first open items that require refrigeration, such as ketchup or salad dressing. That way you'll know when it's time to discard or replace something.

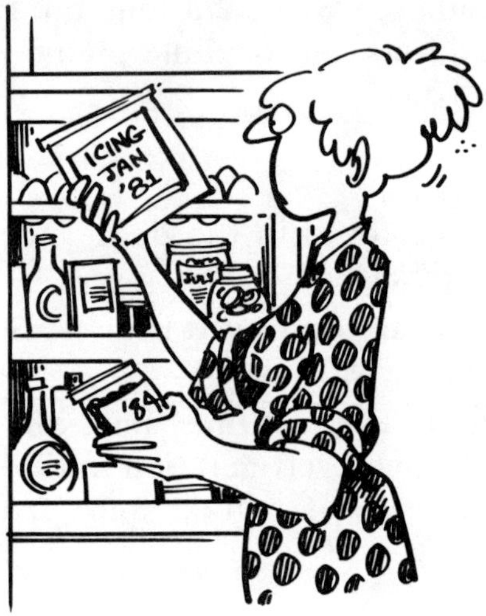

Unripe fruit

- If you want to ripen fruit fast, place it in a paper bag with a piece that's already ripe. The gases from the ripe produce will speed the ripening process in the unripe pieces.
- Underripe tomatoes should not be placed on windowsills to ripen, because sunlight destroys nutrients. Ripen them away from the sun and at room temperature.

Vegetables

- A trick for keeping broccoli, lettuce, cauliflower, and celery fresh is to wash them well, shake off as much water as possible, and store them wrapped in paper towels inside plastic bags.

Cold enough for you?

- Test the gasket of your fridge by closing a dollar bill in the door. If it slips out easily, you need a new one.

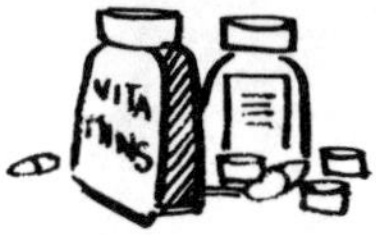

Safe storage tip

- Don't stow salad for a crowd or a big batch of popcorn in a garbage bag. Many are made of plasticized vinyl and the vinyl can "soak" into food, making it unsafe.

Did you know . . .

- Someday you'll be able to buy food by the yard that requires no refrigeration. Already available in Japan is a combination of powdered food and an edible, plastic-like substance. Great for camping trips or places where refrigerator space is limited.

The Conscientious Cook

Relaxing at mealtime

- Don't paint the dining room red. It's a favorite color in restaurants—because it speeds up certain body functions, causes you to eat more and faster, and vacate the table sooner. Not what you want at home.
- Don't bolt your food or you risk indigestion—or worse. The American Red Cross warns that gulping food is a common cause of choking and "café coronaries."

Avoiding the danger from meats

- Very well-cooked beef and pork are high in cancer-causing mutagens, so don't char your food. Three meals of strictly well-cooked meat equal the cancer-causing potential of smoking half a cigarette.
- If you're cutting back on barbecued meat because of reports that food exposed to high heat from charcoal and wood can cause formation of cancer-causing hydrocar-

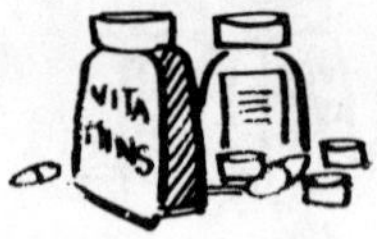

bons, get that outdoor flavor with FDA-approved liquid smoke.

Microwaving pork? Be sure it's cooked

- The pork roast may look done, and your meat thermometer may read 170 degrees, but if you've prepared it in your microwave oven it may still contain dangerous organisms. To be on the safe side, do the following:

  Select roasts smaller than 4½ pounds.

  Cook at a low wattage (50 percent or less).

  Keep roast standing covered with foil, or hold with temperature probe inserted and set for 170 degrees for 10 or more minutes.

  Take temperature readings at several locations to see if the meat is 170 degrees throughout.

  If any part appears pink or red, put the roast back in the microwave.

Broil your fish

- Broiled fish has almost 100 percent of the protein of raw, while baked has 94 percent. Panfried loses 25 percent. Broiling also keeps in more of the B vitamins and trace minerals.
- Rule of thumb for cooking fish: measure at the thickest point and cook 10 minutes for each inch; double that if frozen.

Chicken tips

- You don't need heavy sauces to make chicken taste good. Simply rub with lemon juice before broiling or grilling. It's a great tenderizer and helps bring out the flavor.
- Chicken will be juicy, not dry, if you use tongs to turn it during cooking. A fork will pierce the meat and let the juices run out.

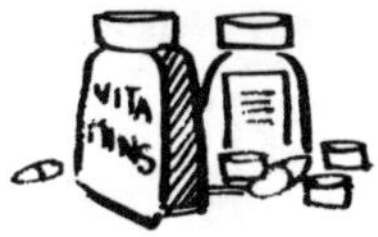

- Test for doneness when roasting or grilling by moving the leg. If it moves easily, the chicken is cooked.
- If you're broiling or frying, pierce chicken with the fork when you think it is cooked enough. If the juices run clear, the chicken is done; if they're pink, put it back on the fire.

Good to the last drop

- Don't toss aside the skin and bones of chicken. Simmer into stock and use it for anything you'd use water for. Fresh vegetables cooked in chicken stock are tastier, more nutritious.
- Or use chicken stock as the base for a quick soup. Add leftover meat and vegetables to the stock, together with noodles or cooked rice.

Keeping nutrients in

- Fewest nutrients are lost in pressure cooking. Steaming's next best. Dry heat processes such as baking and microwave cooking also preserve nutrients.
- Canned foods don't need further cooking. Keep vitamin loss to a minimum by heating only briefly before serving.
- Air breaks down some nutrients, so boil water briefly *before* adding food. The boiling will force the air to escape.
- Don't add baking soda to green vegetables to improve their color. It destroys vitamins.
- Scrub vegetables and cook with their skins on. The fiber in the skins keeps the nutrients in during cooking.
- Slice and chop with a sharp knife. When vegetables are ripped or torn, they may lose nutrients.

Making soup more healthful

- If you're using soup bones, use an acidic ingredient such as tomatoes, vinegar, or lemon juice. The acid will draw the calcium from the bones into the soup.

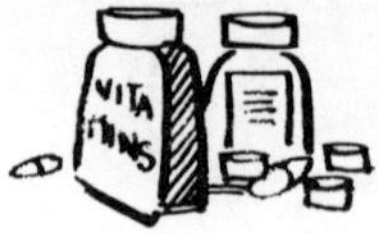

Making a stew

- Cut vegetables into larger chunks and you'll lose less nutrition during cooking.

Cooked or raw?

- Some vegetables are best eaten raw, since they retain more of their vitamins and nutrients. Green beans and salad greens, for example.
- But carrots and spinach make vitamin A more available when cooked.

Is it cooked yet?

- Here's a way to avoid overcooking vegetables. If you can smell the vegetable cooking, it's done.

Steaming vegetables

- Steaming is generally better than boiling. When you steam, cooking water doesn't touch the food, so it doesn't absorb the nutrients.
- Steaming is especially important if you need extra potassium in your diet. Steamed potatoes lose only 3 to 6 percent of the potassium; boil them and you lose 10 to 50 percent. The same holds true for carrots, beans, and peas.

If you do boil vegetables

- Use a minimal amount of water. The more you use, the more vitamins B and C and minerals will be leached into it.
- Save leftover cooking water for up to three days and use it when you're making rice to add nutritional value and flavor.
- Or use leftover cooking water to stretch tomato or vegetable juice.

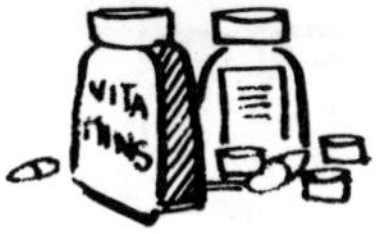

Keep them cool

- Don't reheat leftover vegetables if possible, since reheating increases the loss of nutrients. Instead, add them to salads. Cold cooked broccoli, asparagus, beets, or other vegetables add a nice touch.

More nutritious rice

- Don't wash it before cooking. B vitamins will go down the drain. (Rice marked "coated with glucose and talc" should *always* be washed, however, and is best avoided, since there is some question whether rinsing will remove all the asbestos anyway.)

Dried peas and beans

- You rob dried beans, peas, and lentils of vitamins by soaking them. Instead, boil for two minutes, remove from heat and let stand. One hour of this procedure equals fifteen hours of soaking. Don't rinse.

Don't eat this

- Remove bay leaves used to flavor soup, stew, spaghetti sauce and other dishes before serving. Recent medical reports indicate that bay leaves can be harmful if swallowed.

Flipped over flapjacks?

- Make them more nutritious with whole-grain flour, less sugar, and topping with fruit sauce instead of syrup.

Watch the pot

- Copper pots can destroy vitamins C and E during cooking unless they're well lined.
- But cooking in iron pots is a good idea. Small amounts of iron will be added to your food in the process.

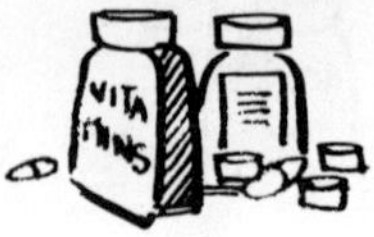

The Main Course: Pointers on Protein

How much is enough?

- The average adult woman requires 44 grams of protein a day (more, if she's pregnant or breast-feeding), the adult man, 56.
- Most American diets contain about 50 grams daily.
- Don't take in more than you need. Excess protein is converted to carbohydrates and fats.
- And, excess protein causes you to lose calcium.

Fish for good health

- If you wondered why nutritionists are always suggesting that you eat fish, you should know that in addition to being low in calories, fish seems to leave you at lower risk for having a heart attack by raising the level of high-density lipoproteins in your blood.

Eating cured meats

- Ham, bacon, and sausage have been linked to cancer because of the nitrosamines that are created when the meat is heated in the factory smoker or your skillet. Adding vitamin C-rich foods (such as orange or tomato juice, or broccoli) to meals of processed meats may inhibit nitrosamines' effects.

Brain food

- Scientists suspect that choline-rich foods (such as liver; also eggs, soybeans) help your memory. (If you serve liver,

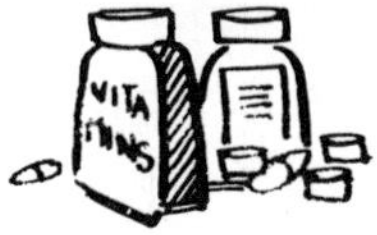

you're sure to remember who in the family doesn't like it!)

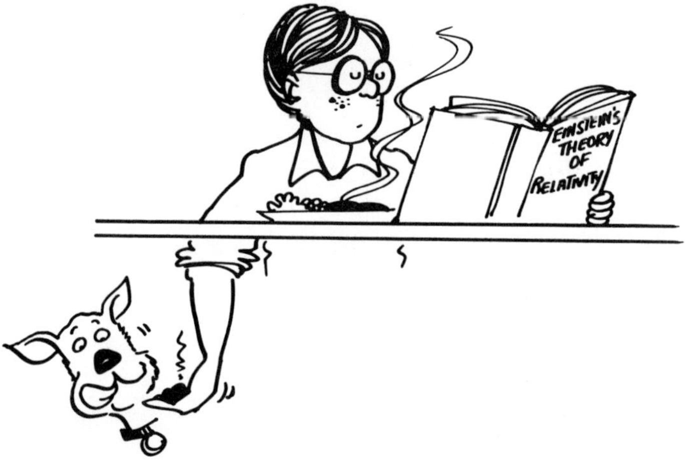

Give eggs a break

- An egg contains 6 grams of high-quality protein, and important vitamins and minerals besides. Unless your doctor has specifically advised it, don't let concern for cholesterol keep you off eggs entirely. Eat two or three a week—and keep your fat intake down by limiting consumption of red meat, whole milk, butter, cheese, and other whole-milk dairy products.

Additional protein sources

- Taking powdered protein may give you more than you need. You can drink a glass of milk or eat a piece of cheese instead—and it's cheaper, too.
- You can substitute vegetable protein for meat protein. Dried beans, lentils and legumes are good sources. But fresh beans and peas aren't mature seeds, so they aren't a good protein source.

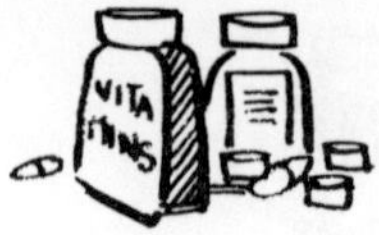

- Certain combinations of vegetable protein or vegetable plus animal protein are low-cost protein sources. Examples are: cereal and milk, macaroni and cheese, tuna-noodle casserole, spaghetti with grated cheese, succotash, peanut butter on whole wheat.

Passion food
- If you're in the mood for romance, avoid the pies and cookies. A high-carbohydrate snack before bedtime will make you feel sleepy. Instead, have a high-protein dinner. Now's the time to go for the caviar.

Side Dishes: Carbohydrates

Getting enough
- Fifty to sixty percent of your total calorie intake should be composed of complex carbohydrates—whole grains, starches, vegetables, and breads.
- If you don't take enough carbohydrates, you won't have energy.
- And if you cut carbohydrates too drastically during a diet, you'll reduce your lean body weight rather than your body fat. That's the opposite of what you want to happen.

Crazy for crackers?
- A yen for breads and other carbohydrates may mean your blood sugar is low, so try eating smaller, more frequent meals throughout the day.

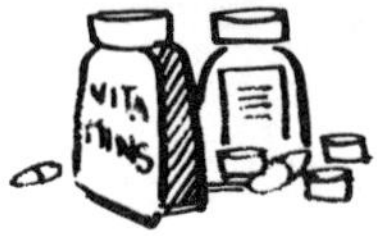

Carrot high

- A Toronto researcher says carrots convert to sugar and get into your bloodstream *faster* than sugar and warns that you shouldn't eat too much of any sugar-boosting food. Sugar from parsnips is the most quickly absorbed, followed by carrots, honey, cornflakes, white rice, whole-wheat bread, instant potatoes, white bread, candy bars, brown rice, raisins, bananas, table sugar, apples, ice cream, yogurt, tomato soup, pasta, baked beans, chickpeas, lentils, and peanuts. (Of course, you'd have to eat a *lot* of carrots to take in the same amount of sugar as in one teaspoon of honey.)

Whole fruit, not just the juice

- If you've been tempted to spend money on expensive juice extractors, save it: you're much better off eating the entire fruit or vegetable. For one thing, it's lower in calories per ounce (half a glass of orange juice has 100 calories, while a whole orange has 80 or less). Also, it contains fiber, which is a necessary part of your diet and helps fill you up.

Whip up a fruit drink

- Frozen fruit juice concentrate mixed with sparkling water in your blender has real zip. (Use the same amount of sparkling water as you would tap water.)

A healthful dessert

- If you always keep a jar of fresh fruit compote in your refrigerator, you'll always have dessert ready. It's easy: Just combine four cups of diced or sliced raw fresh fruit with ¾ cup orange juice or thawed fruit juice concentrate. Vary the fruits according to the season; substitute dried or canned fruit when the fresh fruit harvest is slim. Use as a topping for cottage cheese, yogurt, sponge cake.

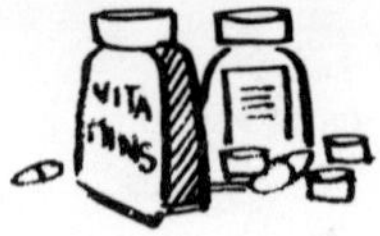

Frozen "pops"

- Fresh green seedless grapes. Eat them like hard candy or let them melt in your mouth.
- Fill a small paper cup with crushed pineapple, fruit juices, or applesauce. Stick in a wooden stick or plastic straw that has been cut in half and freeze.

Super Spuds

- A 6-ounce potato gives you 50 percent of your RDA for vitamin C, 4 grams of protein, fiber, lots of vitamin A—all for just 115 calories!
- Potatoes are a major source of eight essential minerals: sodium, calcium, magnesium, phosphorus, iron, manganese, copper, and sulfur.
- Save the water the potatoes were boiled in, mix with a little powdered milk, and use that to mash the potatoes with. The water is loaded with nutrients and makes milk that is already warm.

The long and short of rice

- Brown rice is better for you than white rice because brown rice retains the grain's natural coating, which has essential nutrients.
- Short-grain brown rice is more nutritious than long-grain because more surface area is exposed, and the additional coating provides more nutrition.

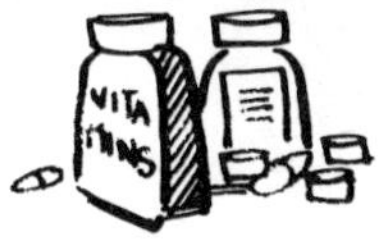

Your Daily Bread: Fiber in Your Diet

Getting enough fiber

- Don't add fiber to your diet by simply taking pills. The idea is to change the *kinds* of foods you eat, not just up your fiber intake.
- Best sources of fiber: bran and bran cereals.
- But you can also get fiber by eating fruits and vegetables, especially peanuts, peanut butter, raisins, bananas, baked beans, frozen peas, canned corn, broccoli.

The best breads

- Whole-grain bread made from stone-ground flour gives you the most nutrients, with 100 percent whole-wheat almost as good.
- Watch out, though: "wheat" on the label doesn't necessarily mean whole wheat. It can refer to regular bleached or processed white wheat flour. Read the label carefully.
- Also investigate when you see the words "brown bread." Some brown bread has little or no whole grain; it gets its color from molasses.

Oatmeal and fiber

- A bowl of cereal has *soluble* fiber that can keep your cholesterol level down by pulling it into the large intestine from which it's eliminated.
- Try no-cook oatmeal. Cover ⅔ cup of old-fashioned or

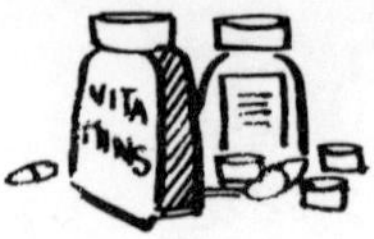

quick-cooking rolled oats with water and soak overnight. Drain the excess water the next morning and try any of these to flavor the cereal: a dash of cinnamon; lemon juice, milk or yogurt; chopped or sliced fruit, nuts or raisins.

Another fiber source

- Dried fruits, nuts, and seeds are high in both vitamins and minerals. They're also dense in calories—not good choices if you're trying to lose weight, but excellent if you're trying to gain.

High-fiber diets

- On a high-fiber diet you need lots of water, especially if you're eating lots of bran. You need about two liters (the amount in a large soda bottle) per day. Keep an empty soda bottle filled with water in the fridge to keep track of your liquid intake.

Cholesterol: Facts About Fat

Which fats are the good ones?

- Most nutritionists suggest that you select polyunsaturates, which reduce cholesterol in your blood, rather than saturates, which increase it. (However, recent evidence indicates that *all* fats may be potentially dangerous.)
- Rule of thumb: The more solid the food at room temperature, the higher it is in saturates. Examples: butter and lard. Vegetable oils, mayonnaise, margarine (percentage varies with brand) are all polyunsaturates.

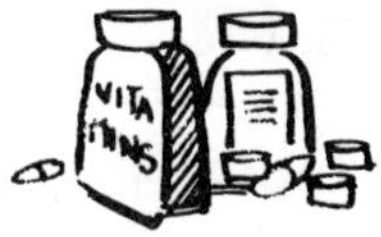

- Monosaturates (like peanuts, olives, olive oil) don't affect your cholesterol.

Controlling fat intake

- Your fat intake should consist of no more than one fourth of the calories you eat each day.
- It's obvious that cream and butter are "fat" foods, but did you know that one third the calories in a bowl of granola and three fourths of a steak's calories are fat calories? You can get a listing of fat calories in 200 common foods if you send $3 to the Center for Science in the Public Interest, Box 43606, Washington, D.C. 20010.

Choosing a margarine

- The label may indicate the ratio of polyunsaturated to saturated oils. Many nutritionists recommend a ratio of at least one to one.

Oily foods that are good for cholesterol

- Oily fish such as salmon, mackerel, tuna, and bluefish are good for you if you're trying to lower your cholesterol. They are high in special fatty acids that make blood clots (one of the problems associated with high cholesterol) less likely to form.
- But shrimp is a high-cholesterol food and shouldn't be eaten more than once or twice a month.

Low-cholesterol cooking

- Substitute margarine for butter or lard.
- Use yogurt rather than sour cream.
- Substitute one egg white and two teaspoons polyunsaturated oil for a whole egg.
- Three tablespoons cocoa powder plus one tablespoon polyunsaturated oil can be substituted for an ounce of baking chocolate.

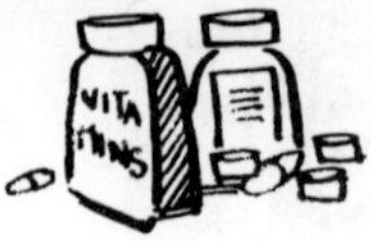

- Substitute skim milk or low-fat cheese for whole-milk cheese.
- Stay away from margarines and vegetable shortenings that have been completely hydrogenated, a process that changes liquid oils into solids. They have become saturated fats.
- Use a vegetable-oil spray to grease pans.
- Avoid lard, salt pork, suet, chicken fat, and products containing coconut oil.
- You can make salad dressing without oil. Try vinegar, lemon juice, low-fat yogurt, or buttermilk as the base. Season with pepper, mustard, horseradish, herbs, and salt in moderation.

Carob vs. chocolate
- Carob, the chocolate substitute sold in health food stores, has less fat than chocolate and no caffeine. But it does have as many calories (114 per tablespoon) and more carbohydrates.
- To use carob in cooking: Substitute one tablespoon carob powder for each tablespoon of cocoa, or three tablespoons carob powder and one tablespoon water for each square of chocolate.

Pass Up the Salt

Yen for salt?
- If you crave salt, you may be under stress. Try adding vitamin C-rich food to your diet.
- If your doctor has advised you to give up salt, you might want to know that it's likely you'll find the first month very

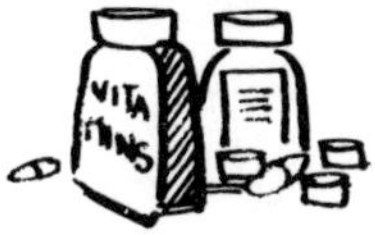

difficult, but after four or five months you will find the taste of salt very unappealing. That's what researchers have found. So hang in there.

Going with the grain

- You need only ¼ gram of salt daily, but up to 5 (about a teaspoon, or 2,132 mg.) is considered safe.
- However, most Americans consume about 24 grams daily—not so much from the shaker, but from processed food. A Big Mac has 1,510 mg., a cup of chicken noodle soup 1,999, a Kentucky Fried Chicken dinner 2,285, a pickle 4″ × 1¾″ 1,928, and a slice of American cheese 322.

Salt by any other name . . .

- Is just as bad for you. If you're cutting your intake, check the label, avoid products with: *baking soda* (in bread), *baking powder* (baked goods), *sodium nitrate* (cured meats), *sodium sulfite* (dried fruits, maraschino cherries), *disodium phosphate* (quick-cooking cereals, processed cheeses), *sodium alginate* (chocolate milk, ice cream), *sodium benzoate* (relishes, sauces, salad dressing), *sodium hydroxide* (ripe olives, certain fruits and vegetables), *sodium propionate* (pasteurized cheese, bread).

Spices that contain salt

- Don't use chili powder and lemon pepper if you're trying to cut your salt intake. They contain salt, as does everything else that has the word "sodium" on the label. (You *can* find these condiments in salt-free form. Try a health food store if your supermarket doesn't carry them.)

Avoiding salt at fast-food restaurants

- Choose hamburgers rather than hot dogs and fried chicken.
- Remove the dill pickle from the burgers.

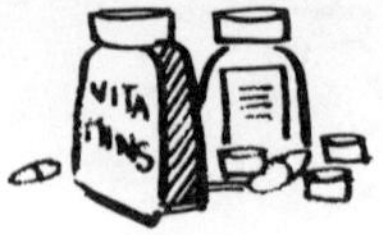

- Pass up the tartar sauce.
- Choose oil and vinegar instead of other salad dressings.

High-sodium vegetables

- If you're watching salt, stay away from these veggies (in increasing order of salt content): frozen cauliflower; frozen broccoli in cheese sauce; frozen brussels sprouts and peas in cream sauce; canned vegetable juice cocktail; canned spinach; frozen carrots in brown sugar; au gratin potatoes; canned tomato sauce, and canned sauerkraut, which has the most salt of all.

Hidden salt in frozen vegetables

- Even vegetables that don't indicate added salt on the label may be high in sodium, since starchy vegetables (such as peas) are sometimes sorted in a salt solution, and others are skinned in a salt solution before freezing.

Salt and microwaving

- Don't add salt before cooking vegetables in a microwave oven. It toughens them.

Low-salt tuna and cottage cheese

- Rinsing regular tuna under tap water in a strainer for 1 minute will wash out almost 80 percent of the sodium, making it comparable to special "salt-free" tuna and much less expensive.
- A minute of rinsing will cut the sodium content of cottage cheese in half. It still tastes better than the "dry-curd" cottage cheese in the dairy section. It's especially good mixed with fruit.

Chapter 2

Here's to the Shape You're In

DIETING

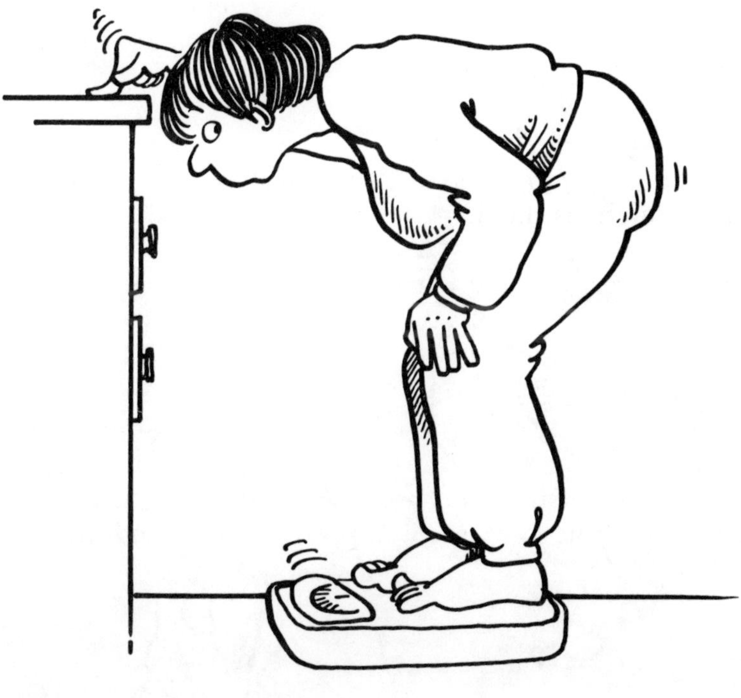

Getting a Good Start

How fat are you?

- Try this at the seashore. (It's more accurate than a pinch test, since it reveals fat that's way under the skin.) Take a deep breath and try to float. If you're only 13 percent fat, you'll sink quickly (even in the ocean); 15 percent, you'll sink slowly; 22 percent, and you'll float while breathing shallowly; 25 percent, and you'll float easily. The last to sink is the fattest. (Results may vary according to age, lung volume, and water temperature.)

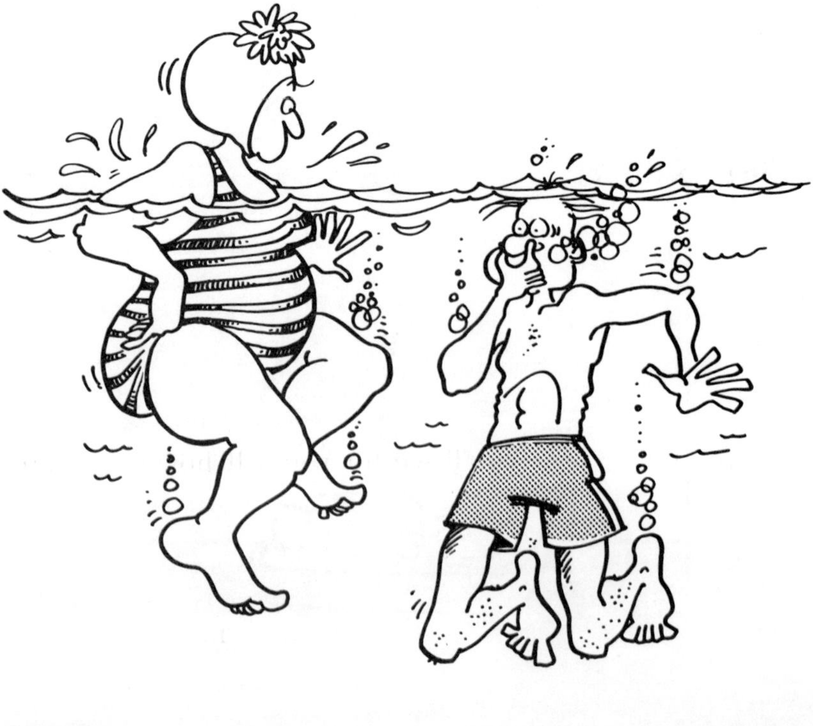

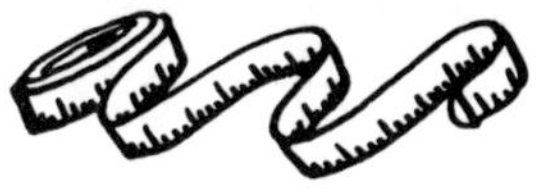

Maybe you're not as fat as you think

- *Glamour* magazine polled 33,000 women between the ages of eighteen and thirty-five to find out what they felt about their weight. Even though 75 percent of them felt they were too fat, only 25 percent actually were overweight. In fact, the study found that more young women are *underweight* than overweight.

Measuring up

- Metropolitan Life Insurance Company says you can deduct two years from your life expectancy for every inch your waistline exceeds your chest.
- Ideally, a man's waist should measure at least six inches less than his chest. A woman (measured just below the bustline) should have the same proportion.

The odds are with you

- Researchers have found that obese people become lean more often than lean people become obese.

Seeing's believing

- Cut eyeholes in a paper bag. Get undressed, stand in front of a mirror, and slip the bag over your head. Your nice makeup job won't distract you from taking a good look at your body—as you've never looked at it before.
- Then, the good news. If you have someone take a photograph of you wearing light clothing against a dark background, you can take a black felt-tip pen and ink out those lumps and bumps. You'll see for yourself how good you can look.

Calvin Klein in time

- A British magazine reports that the one item most women hope to wear after they lose weight is not a bikini, it's jeans.

Make your diet succeed

- Avoid the pitfalls that make people fall off the diet wagon. For one thing, don't choose a diet that's based only on deprivation. Instead, learn a new way to eat. Try lower-calorie meats, fish, fruits, and vegetables that you've never tasted before.
- Follow a balanced program. You'll keep your energy up and feel better—which will give you the strength to stay on your diet.
- Exercise is a must. If you don't make it part of your weight-loss plan, you're treating a symptom (fat) rather than a cause (an inactive lifestyle).

Best time to start

- If you begin a diet right *after* your period, you'll probably do better. Hormones make you feel bloated and constipated before and during—and you may crave sweets and feel lazy.
- Also, you should begin a diet when your life is calm, since dieting itself is stressful. If you're changing a job, ending a love affair, or awaiting an IRS audit, hold off on the dieting. You'll probably do better if you wait till the crisis has passed.

But I hardly eat a thing

- Diet dropouts underestimate how much they eat daily by as much as 50 percent. If you keep a diet diary and enter everything you put in your mouth, you'll know exactly what you're eating—and maybe you'll stop kidding yourself.
- Try putting your food diary in a photo album page and using it as a place mat. It will be a reminder to keep track of what's going into your mouth.

Lose sixteen pounds a year eating corn muffins

- No, this is not a miracle diet, it's a matter of arithmetic. A corn muffin has 220 fewer calories than an almond Danish (130 vs. 350). If you've been eating Danish pastries and switch to corn muffins you save 1,100 calories a week. So, for fifty weeks a year, you save 1,100 calories a week. So, for fifty weeks a year, you save 55,000 calories, or sixteen pounds. Moral: what you eat can count more than how much.
- Since it takes 3,500 calories to add or subtract a pound, you can lose a pound a week by eating 500 fewer calories than you normally would per day. Frozen low-cal entrees, and "lite" substitutes for margarine, salad dressing, jellies, canned fruits, can be big helps.

Supplementing your diet

- Most dieters don't get sufficient iron, magnesium, and zinc. You may be missing other important nutrients, so ask your doctor to recommend supplements.

Diet and medication

- High-protein diets speed the metabolism of some drugs (so they're less effective), and high-carbohydrate diets break down some drugs too slowly (so they accumulate in the body). Unbalanced diets aren't recommended—but if you're on one, you should certainly check with your doctor to make sure you're getting the right medicine dosage.

A friend in need

- Diet with a coworker. Take turns bringing lunch. It saves trouble, makes meals more interesting, and will help you stay on track—especially if you're competitive!

Tricks of the Trade

Sweet vs. sour

- Some tastes clash with each other. Knowing this, perhaps you can make an urge go away. If you want a sweet, chew a lemon. Or drink a glass of diet soda if you yearn for something salty.

Keep it simple

- Don't plan elaborate diet menus. Experimenters have discovered that even rats who are stuffed will eat more if they're offered a new food.

Turn the lights down low

- Snackers in one experiment ate twice as many nuts when they were spotlighted as when they were dimly lit. (Be-

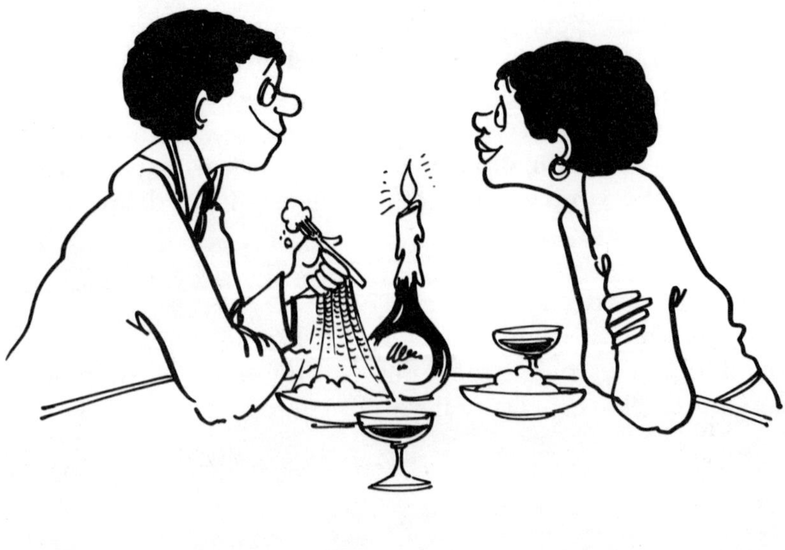

sides, dim lights may lead to romance. And who thinks about food then?)

Depressing your appetite

- Twenty minutes before you eat, have an acidic food or drink like grapefruit or tomato juice. Acids stimulate an intestinal hormone that tells the brain when you're full.
- Or start the meal with a cup of soup (not the creamy kind, of course; broth is best). People who do tend to eat fewer calories at the meal.
- And tighten your belt. It's been established that feeling increased pressure will keep you from eating too much.

On the road

- Don't turn a car trip into a diet disaster. Take along a cooler packed with fruits, vegetables, bottled water, and diet soda.
- And bring your immersion coil to make coffee, tea, bouillon, low-calorie hot chocolate.

A wise dieter eats breakfast

- Penn State scientists found that breakfast skippers are more likely to eat a high-calorie snack later. (Besides, they take in 40 percent less calcium and vitamin C and 10 percent less iron and thiamine than people who do eat breakfast.)
- The fewer meals a person eats, the greater his tendency to obesity, according to research. Obese teen girls in one study actually ate less in crash diet efforts than normal weight girls. But since they were poorly fueled, they were sluggish and spent nearly five hours more a day sleeping or sitting than their thin friends. *That* put the weight on.

Worst time of day for dieters

- More dieters confess to snacking between lunch and dinner than at any other time. After dinner was the second most difficult time, and during cooking was the third. Try to find an activity that will keep you out of the fridge.

Stopping snack attacks

- If you have the urge to eat, force yourself to wait ten minutes. You may find that it will pass.
- Or, quickly drink a large glass of water.
- Treat a snack like a meal. Sit down to eat it, and be sure to record the calorie count in your diet diary.
- Try exercising instead of eating. Sometimes binges are triggered by negative moods which can be lifted through physical activity.

Don't hang out in the kitchen (or you'll hang out everywhere)

- Sampling as you cook can make you fat.

The "just one bite" problem

- Often it's not what you're eating, but the amount that's the problem. Eat one bite each of candied sweet potato (49), bread stuffing (75), giblet gravy (64), creamed onions (28), cranberry sauce (51), pecan pie (115) and you've swallowed 400 calories. On the other hand, you could have chosen a baked potato, followed by ½ cup of ice milk for dessert: half the calories and none of the guilt! Moral: plan what you eat.
- The food you sample as you cook adds up too. A spoonful of fried rice has 70 calories; potato salad, 50. (If you must snack, stick to mushrooms and shredded cabbage: only 2 calories in a spoonful.)
- You'll avoid dipping into tempting ingredients if you store them way in the back of the cupboard out of arm's reach. It sounds so simple it's dopey—but it's true!

Fat vs. sugar

- High fat intake. It's the proportion of fat rather than sugar that determines taste appeal of highly caloric foods. Researchers have found that overweight people often don't like sugar as much as thin people do, but like fatty foods—and a tablespoon of oil is more than twice as fattening as a tablespoon of sugar.

There is no "instant cure"

- Diet pill users, on average, lose only two pounds a month. You can do as well—or better—without them. So avoid possible health risks and save your money.
- Fasting doesn't crash off weight or "clean out" your system. Your weight "loss" is only water; and instead of cleaning out your system, you soon begin to accumulate toxic ketone bodies which put a burden on your kidneys.

Take your time

- If you make sure each meal lasts at least twenty minutes, you'll allow enough time for your body to turn off the hunger alarm. This will prevent overeating.

Dieting in flight

- Airlines prepare low-calorie and other meals suited to special diets. You can even request particular items, such as whole-wheat bread or special vegetables, on certain airlines. Ask when you make reservations.

Small packages

- If you buy or repackage food in individual servings, such as four two-ounce portions of uncooked pasta, or ice cream in half-pint cups, you may cut down your eating. It's harder to stop when you're dipping into a tubful of food.

Did you know . . .

- You can get fat just looking at food. Yale researchers discovered that people looking at, smelling or even listening to a steak sizzle may release extra insulin into their bodies, which helps convert sugar into fat. Solution: stay out of the kitchen, and exercise to encourage your metabolism to do its job well.

Warning signals

- Try marking the calorie count of food on the outside of the package with a wide marking pen. That may prevent your breaking into it in a weak moment.

Imitation desserts

- Stay away from the real thing—and even from low-calorie desserts that just *look* fattening. Researchers have discovered that if it looks and tastes rich enough, low-calorie food may stimulate you to eat. Besides, you're supposed to be learning to live your life without sweets at every meal—and in between.

Pay for it

- Try writing an "adverse check" to keep yourself in line. If you're a Democrat, for example, commit to making a contribution to the Republicans for every week you don't lose a pound.

Beware of the "third-week slump"

- Dieters often lose heart during the third week, when the rapid weight loss of the first two weeks tapers off. Remember—that was mostly water weight. Now the serious stuff is starting to go!

The Diet-Wise Shopper

Don't be a listless dieter

- Shop without a list and you may give in to the urge to buy foods you shouldn't be bringing home. And head for the store after you've eaten: things won't look so tempting then.
- Try trading shopping lists with a friend. You won't load

her market basket with impulse buys you might be tempted to put in your own.

Best calorie "buys"

- You get the most food for 50 calories if you choose one of the following: 18 grapes, ⅓ pound raw mushrooms or carrots, ¼ pound snow peas, 24 radishes.

Diet foods at a glance

- Remember this rule of thumb: food that's thin and watery or fibrous and coarse is lower in calories. But if it's thick, oily, smooth, gooey, concentrated, sweet, or alcoholic—it's calorie-rich.

In the dark about "light" foods?

- No wonder. There are no federal rules regarding the use of the word "light," so one potato chip manufacturer sells a "light" variety that's actually 10 calories more per ounce than the regular type. The label explains that "light" means "light in color"! Some "light" products *are* lower in calories, though. Read labels carefully.

Cheaper means leaner

- The less expensive the meat, the lower the fat content, since heavily marbled steaks are considered prime. The total weight of prime cuts is 40–50 percent fat; choice is 35–40 percent and good has 25–35 percent fat content. "Ground meat," which is made from trimmings, is different. In that case, the more expensive variety (such as ground sirloin) contains the least fat.

Guide to lean meats

- Roasts: leanest include eye or round, shoulder, rump, chuck, sirloin strip.
- Steaks: leanest include flank, round, tenderloin, sirloin tip.
- Ground: round.

• Veal: all except breast.

Sugar by any other name

• Corn syrup, honey, sugar, and other sweeteners may all be listed separately on the label, but they're all sugar. You may be shocked to find how much is in some processed foods, and choose to make your own.

Making Calories Count

Handy measures

• 22 strands of spaghetti, from elbow to wrist in length, are 100 calories.

• A potato the size of an egg has 50 calories.

• A banana the length of wrist to tip of little finger is 60 calories.

• A palm-sized salmon steak, as thick as a thumbtip, is 225 calories.

• A stick of cheddar the size of your ring finger is 100 calories.

• Two heaped tablespoons of peanuts are 140 calories.

• An apple that fits inside two hands at right angles is 50 calories.

Porky's leaner now

• Food scientists have developed pigs that are less fatty, thus less fattening. A three-ounce portion of pork contains 197 calories—the same as a cup of cottage cheese. It is also high in iron, zinc, and the B vitamins.

Saving calories on ground meat

- Grind your own, choosing the leanest cuts. You may want to add a touch of vegetable oil before cooking.
- Cut the calories in meat loaf by placing it on a small cake rack. Then place the rack into a pan. The meat will brown on all sides and the fat will drip off.
- Draining one pound of cooked ground beef removes 290 calories.

Trimming fat calories

- Before cooking meat, trim the fat. If you trim stew meat, you'll put 490 calories into the pot per pound instead of 960.
- The longer you cook fatty meats, the less fat is left. Dieters should order meat medium to well done.
- Make soups and stews a day ahead and refrigerate. Remove congealed fat before you serve them. Each tablespoon you remove means 117 calories less in the serving dish.

Low-calorie cold cuts

- Try the recent newcomers to the grocery case: salami, bologna, hot dogs, and ham made of turkey. They're not only lower in calories than the ones made from beef or pork, but also are cheaper.

Skinning the bird

- Discarding the skin of cooked poultry will cut fat calories in half. Use a paper towel instead of a knife to remove it. The towel grabs much better.

Talking turkey

- The white meat of roasted turkey has about 176 calories per 3½-ounce serving, but the dark meat is 40 percent fattier. (However, the dark meat of chicken is not fattier.)

- Roast turkey and turkey roll have about the same number of calories—but the sodium count, low on the roast turkey, *soars* on the roll. Avoid it if you're cutting back on salt.
- If you remove the skin before cooking, turkey doesn't taste nearly as good. Instead, cut calories by pricking the skin all over before you roast. A lot of the fat will drip off.

Buying poultry

- Here's a rule of thumb: the younger and smaller the bird, the leaner the meat.
- Frozen turkeys are often prebasted, which means they've been injected with oil, butter, or broth. Buy fresh if possible.
- Broilers are 10 percent fat (or less), roasters are 12–18 percent, and large hens are 20–30 percent fat.
- Other lean poultry: Cornish game hen, turkey, pheasant, wild duck, quail.
- Fattiest poultry: domestic duck and geese.

It's all in the cooking

- Here's how the same chicken leg and thigh combination has different calorie counts depending on preparation: raw or poached, 410 calories (165 without the skin); roasted, 290 (190); baked in foil, 340 (195); curried (with skin), 485; deep-fried (with skin), 485.

Calories—foiled again!

- For low-calorie entrees, avoid fats and sauces without eating tasteless food. For example, try wrapping food in foil—the fancy name is cooking *en papillote.* Put fish and a few slivers of fresh vegetable in foil, seal, and bake at 500 degrees for eight minutes, turning package once.
- Other suggestions: salmon and spinach, chicken with scal-

lions and carrots, scallops with snow peas and ginger. However, red meats don't cook well this way, since they don't brown.

Gravy with fewer calories

- Thicken with cornstarch instead of flour. Cornstarch has the same calories as flour but twice the thickening power, so you'll use less.

Fish for dieters to avoid

- Most fish is high in protein, low in fat—except canned salmon, tuna in oil, and sardines. (Tuna packed in water has 20 percent more protein and up to 161 fewer calories per 3½-ounce serving than tuna packed in oil.)
- Shrimp is low in calories, but high in cholesterol.

"Diet" entree prices seem fishy?

- Your "lite" fish sticks may cost more than regular ones because they contain more high-cost fish and less low-cost ingredients like bread.

Slim pickings at the salad bar

- Pass by: bean, macaroni, and potato salads, and mayonnaise. They're all filled with calories.
- Load up on lowest-calorie items: parsley, carrot strips, lettuce, mushrooms, radishes, and onions.
- And avoid those dressings: 124 in a tablespoon of each. Instead, try a sprinkling of grated cheese (25 calories per teaspoon).

Juice vs. fruit?

- If you're choosing a snack, pick the whole fruit, not the juice. It has more fibers and much more bulk for the calories. A whole apple—which takes much longer to eat—has the same calories as ½ cup of juice.

An orange is not an orange is not an orange

- Calorie counts vary. A navel sails in at 89, while Valencia contains 62 and a temple 85. Lower-calorie tangelos (47) and tangerines (39) are tasty, but haven't as much vitamin C.

Canned fruit

- Pouring syrup off canned fruit doesn't remove the sugar—or the sugar calories. Choose juice-packed fruits with no sugar added.
- The liquid from juice-packed fruit is low in calories, high in nutrition. Reserve it and serve as fruit juice or use to make low-calorie gelatin.

Baking your own bread

- Substitute soybean flour (326 calories per cup) for up to one third the amount of all-purpose flour (455 calories per cup) called for in a recipe.
- Invest in an electric slicer so you can make your own super-thin diet bread slices.

Whole-wheat vs. white bread

- Whole-wheat and most common breads have about the same number of calories (60 to 70 per slice). So choose whichever taste you prefer.
- But if you choose a specialty bread, you may be adding quite a few extra calories: bagel (168); small croissant (200); hard roll (160).
- You'll consume the least calories if you select loaf bread that's thin-sliced (around 45 calories).

At the dairy case

- Try buttermilk. Sounds fattening, but it isn't. It used to be what was left after the butterfat was removed from milk. Today it's skim milk that's been cultured, with yellow flecks of fat added. It's low-fat, but it does have added salt.

Watching your spread

- One ounce of butter, at 210 calories, has twice as many as sugar, three times as much as bread, ten times as much as potatoes, and the equivalent of a scoop and a half of ice cream.
- Try cutting down on the amount of butter the recipe requires. You probably won't even notice the difference.
- Don't kid yourself into thinking that margarinc has fewer calories than butter. Both have 9 per gram, about 124 per tablespoon.
- Butter toast when cold and you'll use less. Warm toast absorbs more.

Water for dieters

- Dieters who drink lots of water lose weight better and more consistently than those who don't. (It's worth a few extra rest stops!)
- Try drinking a glass of water when you feel hungry between meals. Doctors have discovered that very often people confuse hunger with thirst.

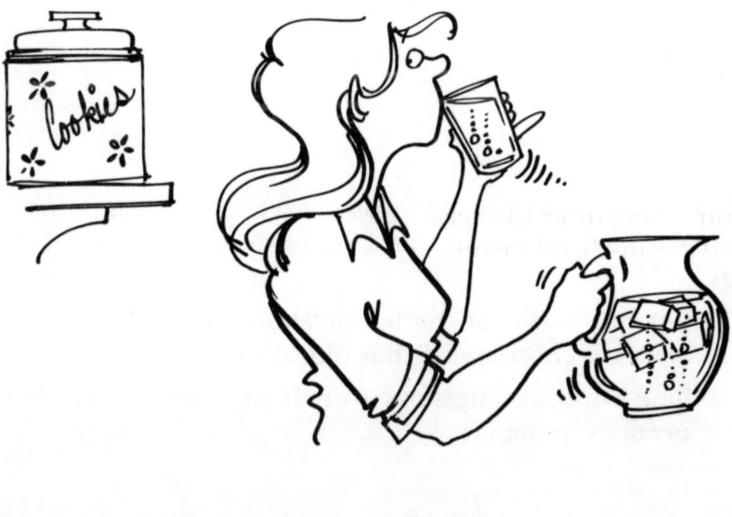

Alcoholic calories

- It's the proof that's important, not how sweet it is. One and a half ounces of 79-proof whiskey is 85 calories. One-hundred-proof whiskey has 125.

If you're dieting and drinking

- You often hear that a glass of wine (75 to 90 calories in 3 ounces) has fewer calories than a cocktail. But some of those oversized wineglasses have much more than 3 ounces—and who stops at just one? Maybe you're the kind of drinker who'd rather have a single gin and tonic or scotch and soda than several glasses of wine.

Beer vs. wine

- Go for the gusto: Beer has around 16 calories per ounce (9 for light), compared to around 25 for wine.
- A 12-ounce serving of beer also has more trace metals, B vitamins, and carbohydrates than a normal serving of wine.

Cooking with Fewer Calories

Chocolate

- Chocolate extract can be substituted for small amounts of chocolate in cold drinks and some desserts to save calories.
- Omit or cut down on butter or shortening when you're cooking with chocolate. It has oils already.
- Combine chocolate desserts with fruit, particularly cherries, oranges, bananas.

- Use less chocolate in artificially sweetened desserts. The bitter overtones of artificial sweeteners will intensify the taste of chocolate.

Eggs

- Use two egg whites instead of one whole egg and save 50 calories.
- Separate eggs, beat the egg whites until stiff, and fold into batter to increase the volume of a dessert.
- Use no-cholesterol egg substitute in place of eggs. You'll save about 45 calories for each egg.

Milk

- Use skim milk instead of whole milk; save 65 calories per cup.
- Use evaporated milk instead of cream; save 735 calories per cup.
- Blender-whip low-fat, part-skim ricotta cheese with skim milk to make a cream substitute in sauces and batters.

Lower-calorie pies

- Cover pies with a lattice of thin crisscrossed pastry strips instead of a solid layer of pie pastry.
- Or cover fruit pie mixtures with layers of phyllo pastry, very lightly brushed with melted butter. It's less fattening than a conventional pie.
- Or make pies with only a single crust and save about 800 calories. Put the crust on the bottom and cover the filling with foil. Or put the crust on top and serve your "pie" cobbler style.
- Roll pie pastry very, very thin. For frozen, ready-to-bake pastry: defrost, cover with waxed paper, roll until 50 percent wider, trim and discard extra pastry.
- Or simply transfer defrosted unbaked pie shells to larger

pans and stretch to fit with fingertips. Then fill with fruit for more servings.

- Try using less sugar than called for, especially if fruit is very sweet.

Wines and spirits

- Boil rum, brandy, wine, or liqueurs before using them in dessert recipes. You'll boil away the alcohol calories, but the taste will remain.
- Substitute rum, brandy, or wine flavorings for the real stuff. You'll save lots of calories.
- Beware of fruit-flavored liqueurs; they carry a double wallop of alcohol and sugar calories. Even when you cook or flame sweet liqueurs, you will not eliminate the sugar calories.

Low-caffeine, low-calorie

- Substitute decaffeinated coffee for the regular kind in desserts; it's less bitter, so you'll need less sugar.

Lower-Calorie Substitutes

For whipped cream

- Pressurized aerosol whipped cream and "light" pressurized whipped cream have more air and fewer calories than whipped cream.
- Use whipped evaporated skim milk instead of whipped cream. Chill milk, bowl, and beaters very well; beat in one tablespoon lemon juice for added firmness; sweeten to taste.
- Or use low-calorie whipped topping mix prepared according to package directions.

For sour cream

- Use plain low-fat yogurt instead of sour cream; save 350 calories per cup.
- Or, blend one cup low-fat cottage cheese, two teaspoons skim milk, and two teaspoons lemon juice.
- Or, blender-whip cottage cheese thinned with buttermilk.
- Or, use sour half-and-half, or low-fat sour dressing.

For cream cheese

- Replace cream cheese with lower-calorie Neufchâtel cheese.
- Blender-whip fresh farmer cheese smooth as a substitute for cream cheese in cheesecakes. Omit lemon juice.
- Or, use cottage cheese, blender-whipped until all graininess disappears.
- Or, try 4 tablespoons corn-oil margarine and 1 cup dry, low-fat cottage cheese.
- Or, use low-fat ("imitation") cream cheese.

For fruit-flavored yogurt

- Fruit-flavored yogurts are high in calories—up to 260 per cup. Make your own by crushing berries (½ cup strawberries = 25 calories) into plain unsweetened yogurt (150 calories a cup) and save 85 calories or more.
- Or, stir a tablespoon or two of defrosted fruit juice concentrate (15 calories per tablespoon) into plain low-fat yogurt.
- Make your own fresh fruit-flavored, soft-serve frozen yogurt in the blender by combining equal amounts of plain unsweetened yogurt and still-frozen unsweetened berries. The resulting blend will be soft and creamy.

For ice cream

- Use store-brand and bargain-priced ice cream. They usually contain less butterfat, calories, and cholesterol.

- Did you know you could buy ice *milk* cake as well as ice *cream* cake at some specialty stores? Try it for the next special occasion.

For nuts only

- Use nutty or crunchy cereals in place of nuts.
- Substitute raisins or other dried fruits for nuts and cut down on sugar in the recipe also.
- Use walnut flavoring in batters to increase nutty taste.
- Put the nuts on top, where you see and taste them first. Result: you use less.
- Use peanut butter in place of part of the shortening, and use fewer nuts.

For coconut

- Use coconut flavoring instead of dried coconut; this will cut down on saturated fat and calories.

For puddings

- Cook and stir fruit juice with cornstarch (two to three tablespoons to two cups juice) for naturally sweet "puddings"—sprinkle with spice, garnish with fruit.

For gelatin

- Substitute one envelope plain gelatin and two cups fruit juice for sugary gelatin mixes. (First, soften the gelatin granules in a little cold fruit juice; then, warm just enough to dissolve completely.)

All shook up

- Frozen unsweetened berries added to fresh skim milk in the blender froth up into a frosty, naturally sweet "milkshake." Good for after school.

Homemade soda

- Make your own diet soda. Use a tablespoon or two of defrosted juice concentrate in each glassful of club soda or seltzer with ice.

Some Sweet Suggestions

Are you starved for affection?

- If you've a yen for ice cream, puddings and other sweets, you're probably looking for emotional comfort. Try pampering yourself with a facial or manicure or treating yourself to a massage, a movie, or anything else (except food) that makes you feel good.

Let them eat cake

- If you must have dessert, choose sponge or angel food cake rather than pound or any other rich cake. Only 20 percent of sponge and angel food cake is fat, while as much as 75 percent of pound cake may be.

Cutting down on sugar

- You can crush ripe berries, simmer them down to a thick consistency, and add a minimum of sugar for homemade "jam" for spread or topping.
- Defrosted juice concentrate (15 calories per tablespoon) can also be used as sugarless jam or sauce.
- Use more vanilla than called for. It increases the sensation of sweetness.
- Add "sweet" spices such as ginger, cardamom, cloves, cinnamon, nutmeg and allspice, and you can cut down on

sugar. They also help give that pretty brown color to pale, sugar-free foods.

- Use the juice from canned fruits packed in their own juice (without added sugar) to sweeten plain yogurt and in other recipes where you need a sweet taste.

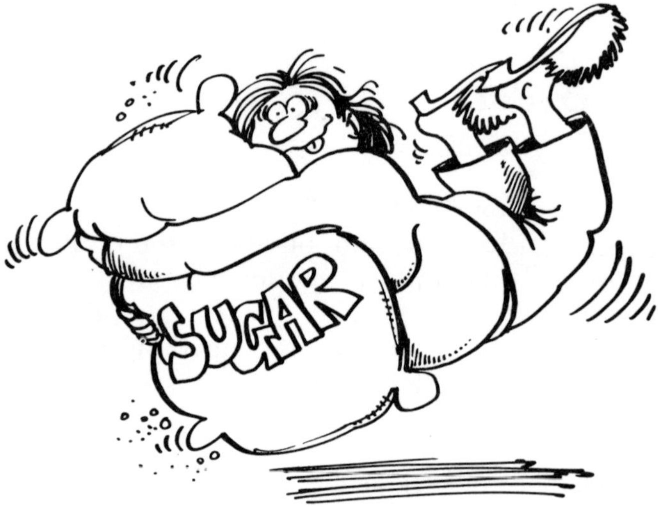

- Overripe fruit is naturally sweeter, and is usually bargain priced. Blender-whip into a fruit puree that you can store in freezer to use as sauce.
- If you reduce the sour and bitter ingredients, you can cut the amount of sugar in a recipe. For example, use less lemon juice in a recipe, or substitute milk chocolate for dark.
- If you boil grapefruit, banana, onions, or tomatoes, or let the water cook out of carrots, you'll caramelize the natural sugars.
- Honey is more caloric than sugar (65 vs. 45 calories a tablespoon), but since it's sweeter you can use less. Replace

a cup of sugar with only half a cup of honey and you've saved 200 calories.

- Granulated fructose (fruit sugar) tastes sweeter than white sugar when you use it on fruit or with acid ingredients. It has the same number of calories as table sugar—but you can substitute ½ to ¾ cup fructose for regular sugar in fruit desserts and save 180 to 360 calories.
- Most fruits taste sweeter when they're fresh and uncooked. (You don't put sugar on a raw apple, but you would add it to a baked apple.)
- A sprinkle of unsweetened coconut over fresh fruit may enhance its sweet taste.

Using sugar substitutes

- "Sorbitol" is intended for diabetics who can't use sugar. It has the same calories as white table sugar, and since it's sweeter you use less.
- If you want to use a sugar substitute, choose recipes calling for less sugar in the first place. You can then substitute less artificial sweetener, and there will be less aftertaste.
- You can make up for the lost volume (from the sugar that's left out) by beating egg whites or yolks until stiff.
- The more baking powder or yeast a recipe calls for, the more it will compensate for the lack of volume from the omitted sugar.
- Dough made by cutting shortening into dry ingredients will be more tender than batter involving the creaming of sugar and other ingredients.
- The main objection to saccharin-sweetened foods is the bitter aftertaste. Avoid it by using saccharin sparingly in sugarless desserts. Once a certain level of sweetness is achieved, additional saccharin will add only bitterness, not sweetness.

- A natural source of unprocessed, refined "fruit sugar" is fruit! Substitute fruit juices, concentrates, fresh and dried fruits for sugar in recipes, and add vitamins and flavor along with their sweetness.
- Both aspartame (a new sugar substitute) and saccharin work best with fruit and fruit-based desserts. In fact, aspartame affects fruit flavors in a way that makes them seem fresher and riper.
- In high heat, saccharin breaks down and becomes bitter instead of sweet. So use saccharin sweeteners in fresh, raw, uncooked desserts, or add it after cooking. If you make pudding, for example, stir in the sweetener after the pudding is removed from the heat.
- Aspartame sweeteners have none of the bitterness of saccharin, but they do tend to break down during high heat or prolonged cooking. There's no aftertaste—but eventually the sweetness simply disappears.
- To help preserve the sweetness of artificially sweetened pies, sprinkle the sweetener between two layers of chilled fruit filling; bake the pie at a higher than usual temperature for a shorter than normal time. This browns the crust quickly without subjecting the filling and sweetener to prolonged high heat.

Dining Out Needn't Do You In

Pointers for menu selection

- Ask the waiter or waitress which foods were prepared from scratch.

- See if you can order a child's portion.
- Have salad dressings and sauces served on the side. Just lightly dip your food into them and you'll get the taste but not the calories.
- Select fish or chicken, not the "dieter's plate" with high-calorie chopped meat.

Did you know . . .

- The standard dieter's plate (burger patty/peach/cottage cheese/tomato) has about the same (or more) calories as the burger and bun. Besides, the bun is a good source of carbohydrates, which will keep you feeling full longer. And you don't need the double portion of protein (from the cottage cheese). So if you'd prefer the bun to the dieter's plate, go ahead and enjoy it.

Best of the fast foods

- Here are the lowest-calorie selections on the menu at some of our favorite fast-food restaurants:
    - Arby's: junior roast beef (250); turkey without dressing (328)
    - Burger King: hamburger (290); junior Whopper (370)
    - Kentucky Fried Chicken: breast with rib (241) or thigh (276); cole slaw (122); potatoes (65)
    - McDonald's: Chicken McNuggets (290); cheeseburger (300)
    - Pizza Hut: ½ pepperoni (430) or beef (490)
    - Wendy's: chili (250); single burger (440)
    - Taco Bell: regular tostada (206), Bellburger (243), Pintos 'n' Cheese (231)

Low-calorie brown-bagging

- Try whipping large-curd cottage cheese in your food processor, mixing it with chopped onion or scallions, thin radishes, parsley and/or sprouts, and eating with melba toast. The Germans call this treat "quark." I call it good.

- Borrow a trick from the Chinese and wrap your meal in a leaf of iceberg lettuce. Spread the leaves with mustard or low-cal mayonnaise, top with thin-sliced chicken, turkey, ham, or beef, or with cheese or vegetables. Roll up and pin with toothpicks.
- Before making a sandwich with a roll, pull out the doughy center. You won't miss it, but you'll save a lot of calories.
- Leftover cooked vegetables are nutritious and a nice change. Toss with low-cal dressing and carry in a plastic storage container. Eat with low-fat cheese and low-calorie crackers for a well-balanced meal.
- You'll keep your lunch crisper if you pack greens and dressings separately and toss just before eating.
- If you're tired of green salad, have pasta for a change. One-half cup of cooked macaroni has only 78 calories. Toss it with a low-cal dressing and add chopped celery and peppers.
- If you eat your "sandwich" in two parts—a scoop of filling on lettuce, plus bread on the side—it will take you longer to eat, and you may find it more satisfying.

Maintaining Your Weight

Bank your calories

- Try to plan ahead. For example, if you cut back 150 calories per day starting November 1, you'll have nearly 3,500 calories (a pound's worth) to eat everything you want on Thanksgiving.

Give yourself a break

- One expert advises that a diet vacation—when you eat whatever you want—is the best way to keep weight off long-term. Some people do it on an occasional weekend, then are *very* careful the following week.

Chapter 3

Here's to Getting a Move On EXERCISE

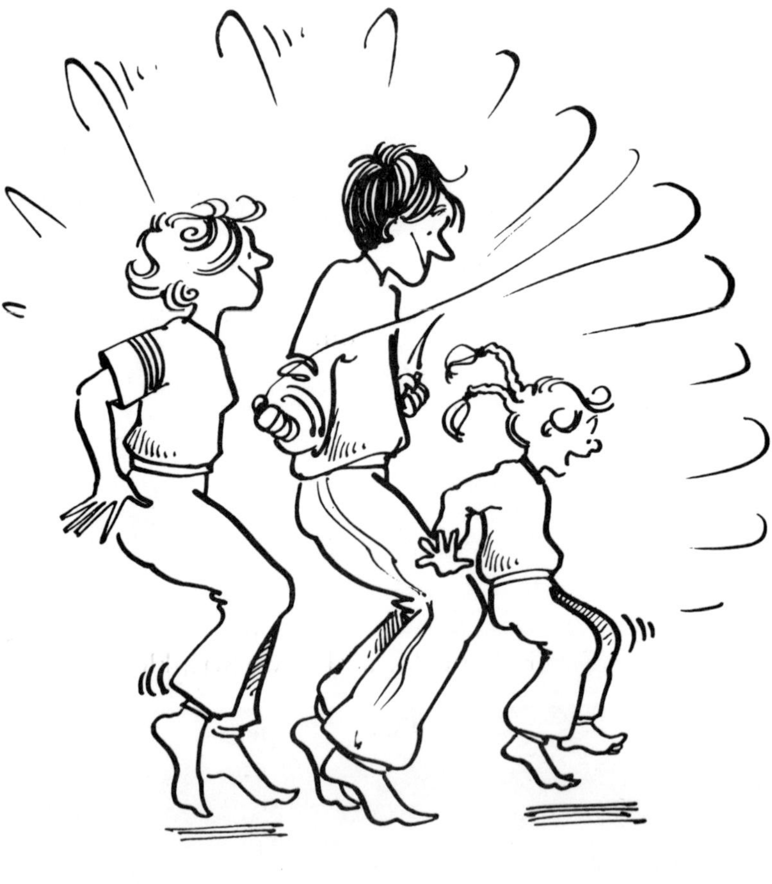

Benefits of Exercise

Keeps you shapely

- Exercise isn't just for the overweight. No matter what you weigh, if you don't exercise you'll begin to exchange muscle for fat. Since fat weighs less than muscle, you may not see the difference on the scales for a while, but you will notice new bulges and bumps.

Calms you down

- Type A personalities are those that are more likely to have heart attacks because of their tendencies to be tense, driven, and anxious. But on a ten-week aerobic exercise program, a group of Type A's aged twenty-five to sixty all showed a decrease in Type A behavior. If it worked for them, it'll probably work for you.

Clears and smooths your skin

- Exercise raises your internal temperature and sends blood to your skin's surface. This brings nutrients to the skin, and keeps it glowing and healthy.
- Regular exercise slows down cell degeneration and breakdown of collagen—the prime causes of wrinkling.
- Studies have shown that older women who exercise regularly have better skin color and fewer wrinkles.

Controls your appetite (and your temper)

- Don't tell yourself that exercise will only make you hungrier. Exercising makes your body produce greater amounts of the hormone beta-endorphin, which reduces your appetite. It also increases your tolerance to pain, counters stress, and improves your mood.

Fights diabetes

- People who exercise regularly may make their bodies more sensitive to insulin and are better able to tolerate foods with sugar.

Improves your mind

- A bout of exercise can increase your mental performance by almost 25 percent.

Lets you eat more

- Lean muscle burns calories, but fat doesn't. A lean, 128-pound woman needs sixteen calories per pound to maintain her body weight; a 200-pound person needs only ten calories per pound. If you exercise, you burn up extra calories—and if you're lean and muscular, your body burns them faster besides.

Lowers your blood pressure

- Exercise can bring on a dramatic decrease in the blood pressure of people suffering from hypertension, with the effect lasting from four to ten hours. Noting this, the *British Medical Journal* recommended a good walk twice daily.

Lowers risk of heart attack

- At the end of a ten-week exercise program (ten minutes of warm-ups followed by thirty to forty minutes of walking, three times a week), volunteers in a Duke University study showed increases in their blood of a substance that helps dissolve blood clots, which may block veins and lead to heart attacks.

Reduces headaches

- Migraine sufferers cut the frequency of their headaches

in half through an exercise program of walking for thirty minutes a day, three days a week.

Saves your marriage

- The healthiest marriages are the ones in which partners exercise together, it was reported at a Woman's Sports Foundation conference. The least likely to succeed are those in which only the wife works out regularly. So—play together and stay together.

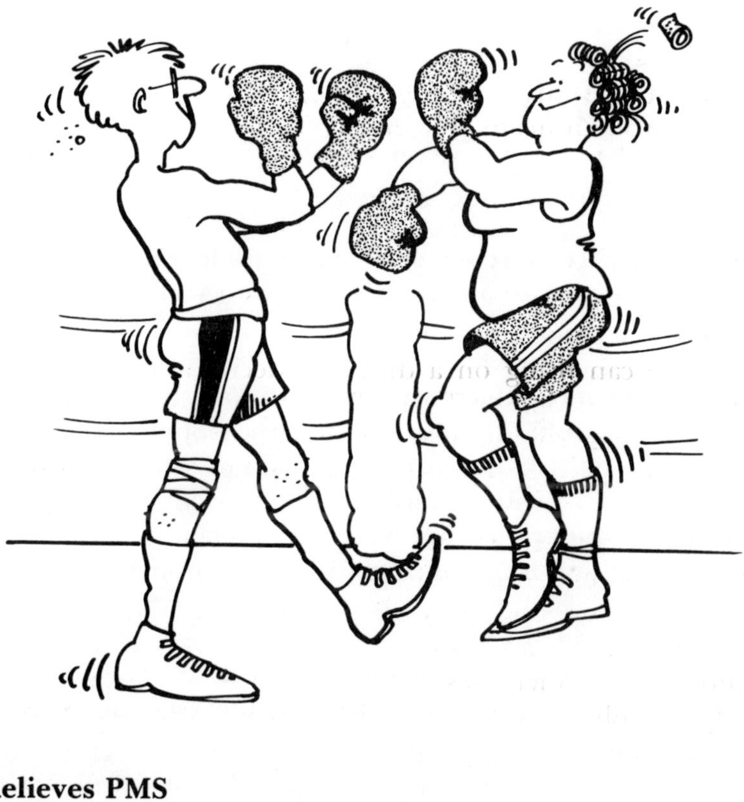

Relieves PMS

- Premenstrual water retention, cramps, and abdominal tension may be aided by regular vigorous exercise such as walking, swimming, or bicycling. Experts aren't sure why, but they believe it has an effect on hormones.

Saves you money

- Some insurance companies offer reduced premiums (up to 50 percent) if you're physically fit. To qualify, you must perform at least a half hour of cardiovascular exercise (running, swimming, or racquetball, for example) three times a week. They may also require an annual physical.

Get Ready, Get Set . . .

Start slowly

- If you haven't exercised since ninth grade, do start slowly. But before you do anything, check with your doctor.

What kind of exercise

- A study of more than 2,500 men showed that those who exercised aerobically more than three hours a week had only half the risk of heart attack of those who engaged in non-aerobic activities. Aerobic activity—walking, running, skipping rope, riding an exercycle, dancing—strengthens your heart and lungs and builds up endurance.

How much to exercise

- To be truly aerobic, an exercise should be done continuously for at least fifteen to twenty minutes without a break.
- Start your exercise program with fifteen to twenty minutes, plus ten minutes of warm-up and cool-down.
- If you want to lose weight, aim for at least thirty to forty-five minutes of continuous exercise. That's when your body

has used up its immediate carbohydrate store and begins to use up its reserve of fat.

How often to exercise

- You might be tempted, but you're not going to get by with just exercising once or twice a week, since it's virtually ineffective.
- Exercising four times a week is three times as effective as exercising three times a week.

How hard to exercise

- Subtract your age from 220 and you'll get your maximum heart rate. Try to get your pulse rate to 70 or 75 percent of that figure during exercise—but check with your doctor to make sure which resting and exercising rates are appropriate for you.

Checking your pulse

- Press the middle three fingers of one hand against the opposite wrist and feel for the pulse. Count the number of beats for six seconds, then multiply that number by ten.

Walk it off

- If you want to counter the effects of a big meal, wait an hour, then walk twenty minutes. If you're in good shape, your body will have speeded up your metabolism (rate of burning food) to take care of the excess calories. You'll get an extra metabolic boost from exercising after the meal.

Keeping fluid

- Contrary to past belief, sports medicine specialists are now recommending that athletes drink plenty of fluids before and during a competition. So if you plan to engage in hard exercise, drink at least half a quart of fluids before, and have a refill about halfway through. Don't use thirst as a guide, since it could be misleading.

Warming Up

Stretch it out

- Don't start your stretching until *after* you've warmed up your tissues with about five minutes of steadily increasing exercise such as walking, jogging, or bicycling. Warmer tissue is more supple, less prone to injury.
- Do your stretches slowly and progressively. Sudden and violent stretching can weaken muscles and possibly damage them.

Don't bounce

- "Bouncing" stretch exercises used to be a standard part of most warm-up routines. However, sports doctors now think this may actually cause muscles to tense up. Slow stretching, using your body weight and gravity, is best.

Eating and cramps

- Forget what your mother told you. You can eat before you swim and you won't get cramps. In fact, long-distance swimmers take nutrition in the water to *prevent* cramping, which comes from energy-starved muscles.

Breathing for exercise

- Try taking a deep breath before you do an exercise or perform a strenuous task such as picking up a heavy bag. Then breathe out while you're doing the work. The job will seem easier.
- Rule of thumb: breathe out on the hard move and in on the easy one.

- Don't hold your breath while exercising. Instead, relax and breathe steadily.

Dressed for Action

Look out for your eyes

- The incidence of eye injuries is highest in racquetball, squash, basketball, soccer, baseball, and hockey. If you play any of these, it's especially important to keep your eyes protected with goggles.
- Many optical companies now offer specially constructed sports goggles, either with clear lenses or ground to your prescription.
- Another option is a heavy-duty frame secured by an elastic headband.
- Eye guards and face masks (which offer even more protection) can be obtained from sporting goods stores.

Go for cotton

- Cotton underwear absorbs perspiration while allowing skin to "breathe." Nylons and synthetics may actually promote infections and rashes, so save them for going out on the town and not on the court.

Cover-ups

- Leg warmers help avoid cramping by keeping muscles warm and relaxed. Wear during both warm-ups and exercises.
- Avoid rubber or plastic "sauna suits." They cause dehydration and deprive the skin of oxygen.

- You need wear warm-up suits only in cool weather or if your exercise room is air-conditioned uncomfortably cool.
- After exercising, let your body cool down naturally, then add clothes to avoid a chill.

These shoes are made for walkin'

- But not if they're tennis shoes, which are designed for flexibility and side-to-side movement. For jogging and walking, you're moving heel to toe in one direction. You need a shoe with a cushioned heel.

Keeping in Motion

Stretch as you vacuum

- Bend one knee in a deep fencer's lunge when you push the wand forward. Straighten up slowly, then bend the

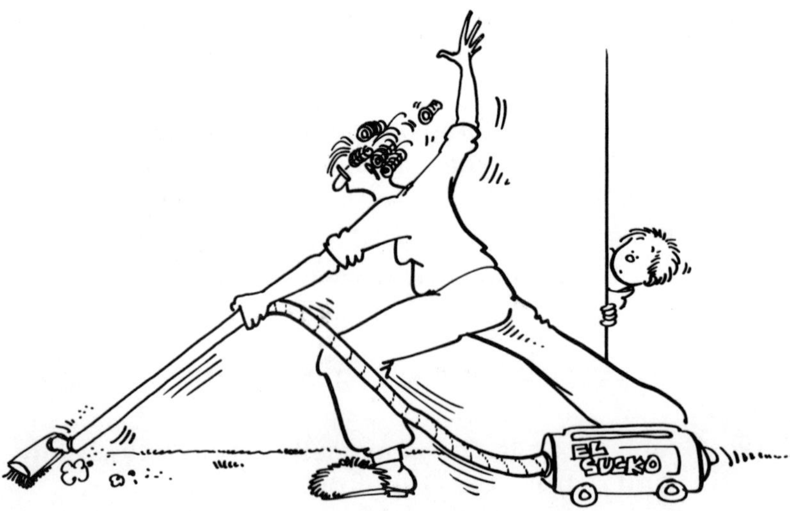

other knee as you make the next forward lunge and pretend you're attacking an enemy. (If it fails to tone you, at least this will help you let off steam.)

On your toes

- Use dishwashing time to help strengthen leg muscles. Just rise up on your toes and lower your heels. Keep repeating until the last dish is in the drainer.

When you're desk-bound

- If you've been sitting too long, relax your body and stretch. Start by spreading knees slightly, dropping head and arms between them. Count five beats, then slowly pull yourself upright using the muscles in your lower back.
- Rotate ankles and wrists for a couple of minutes once or twice hourly.
- Place the palms of your hands on the desktop and slowly lift one leg at a time while keeping your back pressed against the chair. You'll keep stomach muscles firm, reduce lower back pain.
- File the papers yourself instead of handing them to someone else. This may not take off lots of inches, but at least next time you need the file you'll know where it is.

Quick exercise to flex your spine, trim your waist

- Stand with bare feet a foot apart on an uncarpeted area. Extend arms to sides at shoulder level. Very slowly, swing arms, head, and shoulders as far left as comfortable. Then, without stopping, and keeping your feet in place, swing right. The leading arm will come to rest centered almost directly behind you. Work up to twenty swings both night and morning.

Resting your legs

- Try not to stand in one position for a long period. It's hard on knees, bad for circulation, and may cause varicose veins. Best remedy: Keep one foot propped on a small stool or box, and switch legs often.

Lose twelve pounds without dieting

- If you climb two more flights of stairs a day, you'll burn enough calories to lose twelve pounds a year.

For Good Sports

Dance, everybody, dance

- Dancing improves posture, flexibility, strength, endurance, breathing patterns, and agility.
- It quickens reflexes, increases heart efficiency, lowers blood pressure, and improves muscle tone.
- If you're no John Travolta, try folk or other dancing lessons at the Y. They're often offered as adult education.

Maybe golf or baseball is your sport

- If you're cross-dominant (right-handed with a dominant left eye, or vice versa) you have an advantage in golf or baseball. Test yourself: With arms in front of you, touch index fingers and thumbs, forming a triangle. With both eyes open, frame an object in the center. Then open and close one eye. If the object is still in the center, that's the dominant eye.

A pitch for the elderly

- Horseshoe tossing seems to be the ideal exercise for older folks. A tournament provides more walking than a golf game (five miles), and more bending (about 500 times) than tennis doubles. Also, it strengthens hands, wrists, arms, shoulders, and legs.

Good skaters keep up their guard

- Most people protect knees and elbows when skating, but actually half of skating injuries involve the wrist. Hard plastic wrist guards may prevent a fractured wrist.

To strengthen the weakest part of your game

- Wearing a blindfold, practice the movements involved in your sport with the aid of a partner who can watch and evaluate what you're doing. Then, when you find the problem, practice the correct technique blindfolded.

In All Kinds of Weather

Preventing chapping

- Winter or summer, protect lips by coating with a lip balm containing sunscreen, but no zinc oxide.
- Smooth balm on lids, brows, lashes and under eyes, too. Even brow hair can become dehydrated and brittle.
- Also use a moisturizing sunscreen on face.
- For maximum protection, use moisturizer *plus* balm. Allow the first layer to be absorbed by waiting five minutes between applications. And reapply products often.

Wear a hat

- In winter, hats keep heat *in* the body. In summer, a white or light-colored hat reflects the sun's rays and keeps heat *away*.

Symptoms of heat stroke

- If your pulse is faint and rapid, your skin is cold or clammy, or you feel nauseated or faint, get out of the sun. Rest, drink plenty of fluids, and see a doctor if symptoms persist.

Prevent dehydration

- Summer athletes should drink a glass of water every quarter hour during exercise and a glass every twenty minutes for two hours afterward.
- Don't drink caffeine-containing beverages if you want to cool off. And soft drinks aren't as effective as water.

It's not the heat, it's the humidity

- If the thermometer is above 93 degrees F., which is skin temperature, it's not dangerous to exercise if the air is dry. But if it's humid, the air can't absorb moisture. So body heat, which normally leaves your system as sweat, has no place to go.
- When humidity is high, the best exercise is swimming. If water temperature is 83 degrees F. or below, it will absorb body heat.

Sweat it out

- When you're perspiring, don't wipe it off. Sweat's function is to cool your body. Wiping it away only forces your body to work harder to replace it.
- Also, go easy on the sunscreen. Slathering it on from head to toe can interfere with the sweating process by clogging pores. You're better off wearing light, loose clothing that covers you.
- But don't think you're invulnerable to burn even when you're covered up. Fifty percent of the sun's ultraviolet rays can penetrate lightweight, loose clothing. So don't overexpose.

Winter and your waistline

- People with a weight problem gain an average of 7.43 pounds in winter, since appetite increases and people generally become less active. Don't be a winter exercise dropout.
- The good news is that the colder it gets, the more body heat you lose through exercise. So you can cut back a little and get the same results!

Cold weather exercise

- Skier's glasses, with a rubber flap at the top between the glasses and forehead, keep you warm and don't steam up.
- Dress so you won't get wet. Being wet makes you lose body heat.
- Begin in low gear. Don't move up to your normal speed until you've developed some body heat. This keeps you warm but not sweaty.
- Vaseline is a great protection for all exposed areas.
- Vitamin C may help increase skin temperature, and B complex vitamins (brewer's yeast and liver) help your body cope with the cold. Take a vitamin supplement if you suspect you need extra nutrients.
- Ignore the old wives' tale that exercising in cold air will freeze your lungs. Actually, by the time the air gets to the back of your throat it's at body temperature.
- If you can't face the great outdoors, try keeping to your walking schedule in a mall or on an indoor track at a local school.

For winter bikers

- To protect your hands from the wind, put a plastic bread bag over your gloves, fastened with a rubber band. You can tuck a handkerchief under the rubber band, too, for taking swipes at your runny nose.

Other winter sports

- Ice skating is a good exercise only if you do it at a brisk pace.
- When you get ready for downhill or cross-country skiing, don't forget to build up your arms. Pulleys give arms the same backward and forward workout that skiing does and are excellent preparation.

Running and Walking

Walking's the best

- Nothing improves overall health (including circulation) better than brisk walking.
- Brisk walking (3½ to 5 mph) may burn as much as 81 percent of the calories burned in running, and fast walking (5 mph or more) actually burns 100 more calories than jogging at the same rate because you exert more energy taking strides than you do running.
- Walking a mile in twelve minutes burns the same calories as jogging a mile in eight and a half minutes.
- There is only one third of the pressure on the body when walking as compared to running, and less chance of back, joint, and muscle injury.

Walking and cellulite

- Cellulite is just plain fat, and the best way to get rid of it isn't spot exercise but fast walking. The pulling motion of striding helps firm up buttocks and thighs—areas most vulnerable to cellulite.

Are you doing it right?

- You should aim for a pace of at least 3 mph for forty minutes—plus ten minutes of warm-up and ten cooling down.
- Don't bounce up and down. Walk briskly, swing arms naturally, keep your body relaxed—but feel the push.
- And keep at it. The point is to make the exercise continuous, so window-shopping doesn't count (except in your pocketbook, if you're lured inside the store).

If you live in the city

- Protect yourself from air pollution at least to some degree by exercising early in the day or late in the evening.
- Or see if there is a special runner's path or an indoor track you can use to walk on.

Be your own buddy

- You don't have to find a friend to walk with. You actually may get additional benefits from walking if you use the time to unwind, set your own pace, and go on your own schedule. Alone, you may actually enjoy a more productive, unpressured workout.
- You certainly won't be on the streets alone. The U.S. Census reports that walking is America's favorite exercise.

Did you know?

- Over five million Americans save money and stay fit walking to work. Champion walkers are San Diego workers. Nearly 5 percent hoof it to work, followed by New York with 4.4 percent.

For the runners among us

- If you're a beginner and can't run for fifteen minutes, try alternating running and walking. Run for one minute, walk for two. As you improve, reverse the amount of time spent running and walking. Soon you'll be going the distance.

- Jogging in smog-filled cities for half an hour fills your lungs with as much carbon monoxide as a half pack of cigarettes. Try to find a runner's path away from city traffic, or an indoor track.
- Running on the beach is strictly for the soft-drink commercials. If you're doing it for sport, wear shoes to absorb the shocks and to keep your heels from sinking, which may cause pain in heels and lower legs.

Run into the wind

- If you're jogging in winter, you should start by running with the wind so your body gets warm faster. On the way back, when you're overheated and sweating, you'll want to run against the wind.

Other Aerobic Exercises

Jumping for joy

- Jumping rope is probably the most convenient exercise, since you can do it right at home. It's certainly the most efficient. Ten minutes of jumping equals thirty minutes of jogging.
- If you're older or out of shape, try jumping one foot at a time for an easier pace.
- Trying to increase the benefit of jumping rope? Don't do it by jumping faster. Just lift your feet higher.

Exercycle-bored?

- Try switching gears at two- to three-minute intervals. Drop into low gear and work your leg muscles for three minutes, then flip into high and pedal rapidly. Breaking up your exercise this way will make it go faster because you're dealing with five-minute blocks of time instead of twenty.

- Or treat yourself to the Aerobics Joystick (Suncom, Inc.) that clips onto your bike and links it with your Atari or Sears home video game system. The faster you pedal, the faster the game moves. (Buy it at video-game and exercise equipment stores.)
- Or, buy a reading rack for your exercise bike. While you're giving your body a workout, work out your mind—or relax it with an escapist novel.
- And you can always pass the time by watching TV. Just be sure to keep pedaling—even during the exciting moments.

Get in the swim

- If you have back, knee, or ankle problems, you might find that swimming's the remedy. Ask your doctor. Swimming's an all-around conditioner, and the buoyancy of the water relieves stress on injured joints.
- Want to tone muscles? Work against water resistance: Firm up legs by hanging on to edge of the pool, standing on one leg and kicking the other to the front, side, and back; alternate with the other leg and repeat several times. To tone hips, thighs, and bottom, grab a flutterboard and swim laps, using kicks only.

For total fitness

- Aerobic exercise doesn't improve muscle tone or strengthen you. You may need calisthenics or light weight lifting to work on your arms, back, and chest as well as abdominals, waist, rear, hips, thighs, and legs.
- You won't look like Conan the Barbarian if you lift weights. Bulging muscles developed through exercise are the re-

sult of male sex hormones, which women also have but in much lower levels than men. Women weight lifters may have well-defined muscles because of the loss of some body fat.

- If you don't want to invest in weights, instead use two-gallon milk jugs partially filled with water. (Increase the amount of water as you work up to heavier weights.) Tone arms by holding them parallel to your body, then lifting over your head.
- If you're a beginner, use light weights and multiple repetitions. As you grow stronger, increase the weight gradually rather than increasing the number of repetitions.
- If you go in for Nautilus or Universal weight-lifting machines, don't use them any more or less than three times a week. Overuse, especially at first, can cause muscle strain.

Cooling Down

Stretch after exercising

- Strenuous exercise causes muscles to tighten up from stress, and they can tear easily. If you limber up before and stretch afterward, you're less likely to be stiff. Don't bounce or move quickly, but use slow, stretching movements.

Wait before showering

- Your body keeps sweating after exercise. If you don't cool down for at least ten minutes before you jump into the shower, you'll continue to sweat during the shower, possibly even afterward. (By the way, perspiration is odorless. Body odor comes from sweat mixed with bacteria, which a shower washes away.)

Replacing lost fluid

- If you're short of water, you may get muscle weakness and cramping.
- Weigh yourself before and after exercising. For every pound you've sweated off, drink two cups of water.

Easing the Pains

"Morning-after" exercise aches

- Sore muscles eight to forty-eight hours after exercise are probably the result of exercising hard without a proper warm-up. You can avoid them by warming up with stretches. Don't bounce, lift, or jerk limbs: that may make the problem worse.
- And if you take little rest intervals during exercise, you're less likely to be sore. But don't take them during aerobic exercise, which should be continuous.

To relieve muscle cramp

- Stop exercising, massage the area, then slowly stretch the muscles.
- If your legs or calves cramp up while exercising, you may need more potassium in your diet. Bananas are loaded with it; potatoes are high, too. Eat them frequently.

RICE for sprains

- Rest, Ice, Compression, Elevation—the RICE cure—is the remedy for a turned ankle or twisted knee.
- Apply an ice pack for twenty to thirty minutes every couple of hours. In between, wrap the area snugly with an elastic bandage to help reduce swelling. (Be sure the wrap

is tighter below the joint or bruise, and looser on top, so blood is forced to the heat and excess fluid is forced away from the injury.)

- Keep the injury elevated—above the level of your heart, if possible.

Homemade ice pack

- Try freezing water in a foam cup, then peeling off a bit of cup to expose ice directly to the area that needs it. (Be sure and keep the ice moving around the sore spot, or you may get ice "burn.")
- Or try a bag of frozen vegetables. It molds to the body and is fairly sturdy.
- Or use a plastic glove filled with ice cubes.
- Or use a plastic bag filled with cubes.

Cure for a blister

- Prick it with a sterilized needle, drain, and apply a dressing soaked in salt water or Epsom salts. Then paint with gentian violet (from your drugstore), which will dry it and reduce the chance of infection. Apply it three or more times a day. You'll either love or hate the purple on your heel—but it'll be gone within a week, along with the scab.

Hang in There

Sticking with it

- Schedule your exercise at a convenient time and you'll be more likely to do it.
- Vary your routine—aerobics alternated with strength-

building exercises, for example—to help keep yourself from getting bored.

- Try exercising to music. A radio or cassette player with headset is a great incentive to the walker.

Try joining a crowd

- If you like competition, or you don't want to be responsible for your own exercise and want someone else to be in charge, try joining an exercise class. Many Y's, for example, have aerobics classes which you may pay for and attend without paying the fee for a complete Y membership.

Taking it to the limit

- All older folks who exercise are healthier than sedentary types, but competitive types have an extra edge. Elderly joggers who continue to train for competition age far more slowly than those who exercise casually.
- The exercising repetitions that come *after* you are ready to give up are the ones that increase muscle size and strength. Knowing that may help you keep going.

Use it or lose it

- If you have a minor injury, don't give up your exercising completely or you may destroy months of work getting in shape. Rest the turned ankle or pulled leg muscle, but when the worst is over (a couple of days or so) try to follow a limited workout routine, perhaps with calisthenics or swimming. Check with your doctor.

Backsliding is dangerous

- Experimenters found that rats who exercised regularly for six weeks became leaner and their fat cells shrank. But when they stopped, within three days they began eating more than when they were exercising—and more than other rats who didn't exercise at all.

Did You Know . . .

Where to take a hike

- If you don't know where to go, try contacting your local Boy or Girl Scouts, the Y, the Parks & Recreation Department or your city government. Any or all may have historic or nature walks mapped out.

High-protein diet and exercise

- Don't limit your carbohydrate intake severely if you exercise regularly. You need carbohydrates for energy.

Which exercises help you sleep

- Vigorous exercise late in the day keeps you up. But static exercise (push-ups, weight lifting) two hours before bedtime may be your ticket to the Land of Nod.

Is sex good exercise?

- The average man uses four to six calories a minute during intercourse, which is about the same as taking a walk around the block. Of course, we're talking about the *average* man.

How to tell if you're well balanced

- To pass the civilian pilot medical exam, you must be able to stand with feet together without swaying for ten seconds with your eyes closed.
- And (also with eyes closed) hold your arms straight out at shoulder height and touch your toes with alternating hands.

- Military pilots must be able to do all of the above, plus walk a perfectly straight line with eyes closed, and do ten or twelve knee bends.

The healthiest habits

- If you're exercising regularly, you're observing one of the seven habits that the healthiest people keep. The others are: sleeping seven to eight hours nightly; eating breakfast regularly; not eating between meals; maintaining proper weight; exercising regularly; drinking moderately or not at all; and not smoking.

Chapter 4

Here's to a Beautiful You
BEAUTY

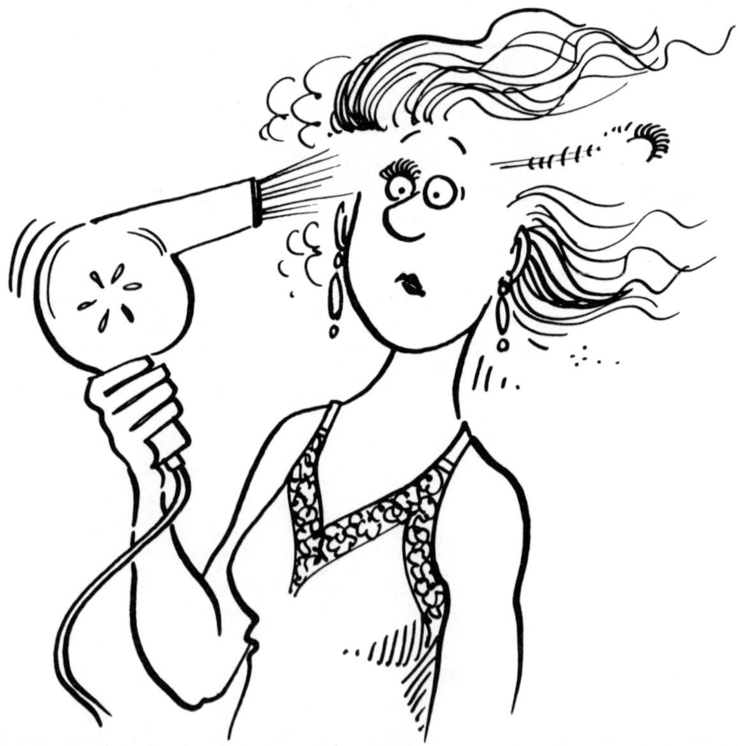

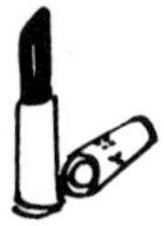

Your Skin and Face

Keeping skin young

- Yo-yo dieting is a no-no: It stretches and relaxes skin, increasing the chance of wrinkles and sags. So try to keep your weight constant.
- Find a way to release tension (warm bath, yoga, exercise) since it can cut off circulation and "set" lines in your face.
- Wear a sunscreen. It'll prevent pigment changes and brown spots and keep your skin from aging.
- Stay out of the sun between 11:30 A.M. and 2 P.M.
- Exercise to get your circulation going. That helps create new skin cells, keeps color in your cheeks.
- Rest, or your skin won't get fresh oxygen and nutrition.
- Don't overindulge. Alcohol is dehydrating, dilates blood vessels, creating that "Rudolph the Reindeer" nose.
- Use extra moisturizer when the room is steam-heated or air-conditioned. Both dry your skin.

Free conditioners

- Drinking six to eight glasses of water a day—*not* including sugary sodas or salty vegetable drinks—to replace what your body eliminates will do more for your skin than any commercial product. (If you drink lots of soda or vegetable juice, you need even more water.)
- Also, since physical activity brings blood to the skin, releasing sweat and carrying nutrients and oxygen, it helps keep skin looking great.

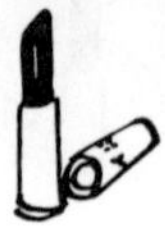

Skin food

- Vitamin A-rich foods (carrots, spinach, sweet potatoes are among them) help keep your complexion healthy and glowing. If it's not, maybe you need more vegetables in your life.

Sunlamps, tanning booths, and your skin

- Ultraviolet B (UVB) radiation can cause premature aging and cataracts, as well as increasing the danger of skin cancer.
- And ultraviolet A (UVA) is not absolutely certified safe, according to the American Academy of Dermatology. Use with caution.
- If you're using acne medicine that contains retinoic acid (a form of vitamin A), you should know that when combined with ultraviolet rays, it increases the risk of skin cancer.

Smoking and your skin

- Carbon monoxide in smoke impedes circulation.
- The burning paper kills new skin cells and causes aging.
- Nicotine may cause brown splotches.
- The drying effects of smoke create wrinkles.

Skin types

- Unsure whether your skin's dry or oily? Blend together juice of one lemon, ½ cup distilled water, one teaspoon olive oil, and three ice cubes. Let sit until cubes are melted. Then apply to thoroughly cleansed face and wait three hours.
- Dampen one cotton ball in the solution and gently wipe across forehead. Wipe a second cotton ball over your nose, and a third on your chin.

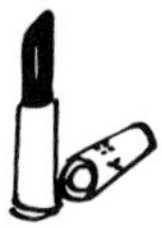

- If all are clean, your skin is dry. If they're dark, your skin is oily. If they're slightly soiled, you've got a combination.

Don't spot-treat your skin

- If you've got a mixed bag of skin problems, the newest thinking is that you should use a salicylic-acid product (for blackheads and whiteheads) in the morning and benzoyl-peroxide lotion (for small pimples and under-the-skin cysts) at night rather than spot-treating. (If self-treating after a month doesn't help, visit your skin doctor.)

Oily skin with dry patches

- People with oily skin or acne should avoid moisturizers. If you must use one to treat dry patches, find one with minimal oil or you'll make your skin problem worse.

To pick a moisturizer

- Test moisturizer by seeing whether it feels hot or cold. Moisturizer for oily skin should evaporate quickly, which would leave your skin feeling cool. Dry-skin moisturizer should feel warm, because it should stay on the skin surface.

Skin chapped? Go green

- Green-tinted moisturizer helps cover up red skin (from chapping, colds), while mauve helps disguise yellowish or tan patches, like freckles.

Nature's moisturizer

- This is great for those who are allergic to commercial moisturizers: Beat an egg yolk, add ½ cup milk and mashed half of a ripe avocado, and blend. You've got a natural cleansing cream and moisturizer for your face. Massage in well, and rinse thoroughly.

Special potions

- Eye creams and other concoctions for specific areas are more expensive because they're more complicated to make. But in the long run they may be more economical, since they'll last a long time because they're concentrated and you use them only on small areas.

"Hands off" your face

- Hands come in contact with more germs and bacteria than any other part of your body. If you are in the habit of picking, playing with, or resting your face in your hands, you're transferring these germs to your face. Break the habit and watch the results.

Cleaning your face

- Doctors recommend using white facial tissues, since the dye from colored ones may irritate your eyes.
- Cotton balls are better for removing makeup than bathroom tissue, which is made from wood pulp and may be harsh.
- Also, vegetable shortening is an effective makeup remover. Massage it into skin and wipe off with tissue.
- Too-hot water can break capillaries around nose and cheeks, causing spidery red lines to appear on cheeks and nose. So wash up with warm water.

Choosing soap

- The most common test of mildness is how easily and thoroughly a soap rinses off. (Exceptions: deodorant and superfatted soaps must leave a residue.)
- Among the mildest: Neutrogena, followed by Aveeno, Alpha Keri, Basis. Not so mild: Zest, Safeguard, and (surprise!) Ivory.

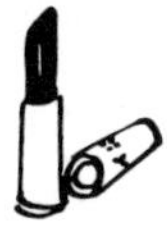

- Scented and deodorant soaps shouldn't be used on your face. They may irritate your skin.

A natural scrub

- Mix equal quantities of cornmeal and regular (not instant) oatmeal with hot water to make a paste. Apply while still warm. Leave on ten minutes. Rinse off with cool water. For extra cleansing and tightening, add a few drops of spirits of camphor to the rinse water.

Toning tips

- Make a mask of buttermilk (or a cup of whole milk with a teaspooon of lemon juice). Pat on, let dry, and then rinse with cold water. This has the proper acid-alkaline balance and works as an astringent.
- If your face feels tight after being washed with soap and water, measure a teaspoon or two of apple cider vinegar into a basin of cool water for a final rinse.
- Here's a pleasant homemade astringent. Mix a teaspoon each of mint, sage, lavender, and rosemary into a quart of vinegar and let marinate for two days. Then strain off the herbs and boil the solution with an equal amount of water. When it's cooled, it's ready for use.
- Or try ordinary witch hazel. It may be as effective as any of the costlier products. Store in a pretty bottle on your cosmetic shelf.

"Scentsitive" skin

- Be careful when you buy an "unscented" product if you're allergic to perfume. Unscented doesn't necessarily mean fragrance free—some small amount of fragrance may have been added to mask the chemical smell.

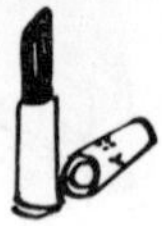

Natural skin cleaner for sensitive skin

- Try almond oil, available at health food stores. Pour a capful into your palm and spread lightly over skin. Rinse and pat dry.

Makeup for problem skin

- An oil-based foundation or moisturizer can contribute to an acne problem by clogging overactive pores. You might be better off with a water-based moisturizer.

Quick cover-up for acne

- Tiny acne scars can be hidden by applying a dot of concealing cream with a pointed brush before you put on your foundation.
- To help heal a pimple, rub a styptic pencil on it three times a day.

Most makeup for your money

- If your mascara has dried up, hold the closed tube under hot running water for a few minutes. The mascara will soften and squeeze out easily.
- When applying mascara, just pull the wand straight out without sliding it in and out of the bottle. Otherwise, air will get into the bottle and dry it out.
- Put lipstick and eyeliner pencils in the freezer before sharpening: you'll get a sharp point without the waste.
- If your blushing powder has broken, don't throw it out. Crumble it up and keep in a small, wide-mouthed jar.
- Don't buy an expensive makeup brush: Use a high-quality artist's brush.

Relieving cold sores

- If you feel a cold sore coming on, rub a cut lemon over the affected area several times a day. This will nip it in the bud.

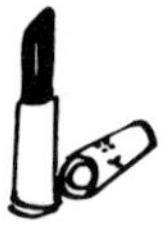

- But if you find yourself with a cold sore, ease the pain by dabbing on spirits of camphor (available at drugstores). If sores persist, you should visit a dermatologist for a diagnosis (cold sores are common symptoms of herpes) and prescription.

Put on a happy face

- If you have to make a public appearance after a crying jag, try using a gentle cleaner. Tears irritate sensitive skin, and rubbing only makes it worse.
- Rinse with cool water, or wrap an ice cube in a washcloth and apply to puffy areas.
- If you've got a moment, lie down and place cotton pads moistened with witch hazel on your eyelids.
- Drum fingertips under eyes, lightly press inside corners of eyes.
- Use a concealing stick under eyes.
- Eyes lined with blue or mauve pencil make whites look whiter.

To lift or not to lift

- Thinking of a face-lift? Lie flat on your back on the bed and hold a mirror above your face. Gravity will cause all that loose skin to fall back, and you will see approximately what you would look like after a lift. If the change doesn't seem dramatic enough, you may want to forgo surgery and put your money in a retirement fund instead!

If your cheek color tends to fade

- Try using the same color in both powdered and cream or liquid forms. Apply the cream or liquid over regular makeup base, then dust over it with powdered rouge.

Smooth idea for chapped lips

- Try pure lanolin, available at your drugstore. It's cheap,

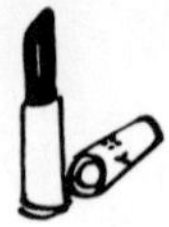

and an application before bedtime may even last through the next day.

To keep your lipstick *on*

- Try applying an ice cube over it. It will "set" the color.
- Or apply a coat of lipstick, followed by gloss, with lipstick on top. This should help the color stay on.

Cleaning a lip brush

- Before dipping it into a new color, dip it in a bit of alcohol poured into your palm. Then blot it before using.

Hot lips

- Wetting lips with saliva makes a lip sunburn worse.
- Since lips burn easily, use a lip balm with sunscreen. (Leave it on five minutes, wipe off excess and then apply gloss.)

The Eyes Have It

A thorough eye exam should include:

- Your medical history, including allergies, medication you're taking
- Exam to check tear flow
- Check for the surface health of your cornea and its curve and diameter
- Internal exam with ophthalmoscope
- Eyelid health check
- Tests for glaucoma and eye coordination

Choosing the right sunglasses

- Pick a frame style that's different from the shape of your face.
- A keyhole bridge makes a big nose look bigger.
- Brows should show above frame or through lenses.
- Dark color at the bottom shortens the face, soft color or none at all lengthens.

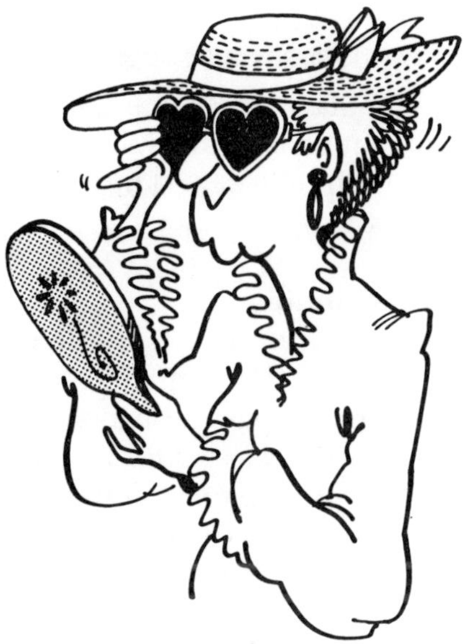

- The bow is most flattering if it's positioned at the top corners of the lens frames, unless your face is long.

What every movie star knows

- Try on sunglasses while looking in the mirror. If you can still see your eyes, they're not dark enough. (You need 30 percent light transmission in average sunlight, 15 percent when in glare.)

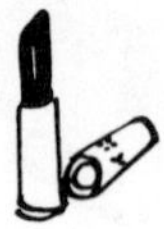

To test the quality of sunglasses

- Holding the sunglasses about ten inches from your eyes, look at a square edge. When you move the glasses from side to side, the image shouldn't wiggle.

Sunglasses in the snow

- If you're on the ski slopes and your eyes start burning, watering, or reddening, go immediately into a dark room. You might be suffering from snow blindness caused by the glare of the sun against the snow. You'll be less likely to get it if you wear sunglasses or goggles.
- You may want to use glass rather than plastic lenses in your sunglasses to avoid snow blindness, caused by short-wave ultraviolet burns of the cornea. The rays can penetrate plastic, but not glass.

Contact lenses and swimming

- Don't push the panic button if you suddenly get a pain in your eyes when you're swimming while wearing soft contact lenses. The simple explanation may be that the lens has changed shape in the water and is squeezing the eyeball. Just put some of your regular wetting solution in your eyes, and you'll be back to normal in three to four minutes.

Glasses overboard

- You can now buy plastic floats that attach to the temples of your eyeglasses so they won't sink if you lose them sailing or boating.
- Prescription swim goggles are also available. Ask your eye doctor.

Men *do* make passes at girls who wear glasses

- Especially if they look terrific. If you use a bit of blush above your eyebrows, you'll give your face a lift.

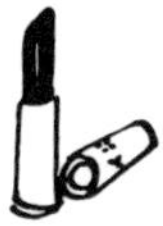

Moisturizing the eye area

- Don't use an all-purpose moisturizer around your eyes. It may cause puffiness and water retention. Use special eye creams instead.
- If commercial eye creams make your eyes swell, try the solution recommended by some plastic surgeons: castor oil. It's non-allergenic, and it works. Apply the oil gently. Blot off after ten minutes.

Mistake-proof mascara application

- Look down into the mirror. Coat the top lashes with mascara first, then apply to lower ones.

Which comes first: lenses or liner?

- Wearers of soft contact lenses should put them in before making up eyes to prevent any makeup getting on them. Avoid lining inside eyelids or using "long lash" mascara.

To prevent streaky eyeshadow

- Pat the crease above your lid with non-alcoholic toner to remove any oil or perspiration before you apply shadow.

Eye-shadow application

- Your eye shadow will stay on better if you put the cream on first, then dust with powdered shadow of the same color.

Ouchless tweezing

- Anesthetize your brows by pressing an ice cube over them for a few moments before you pluck.
- Or, hold the eyebrow between the thumb and index finger and roll firmly for fifteen minutes to numb the area.
- Or, numb eyebrows by applying a baby product used to numb the gums when a baby is teething.
- Lightly buff the tips of a dull tweezers with a nail file, emery board or pumice stone. They'll sharpen right up.

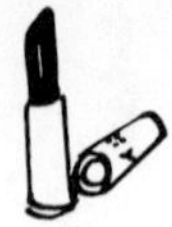

Optical illusions

- You'll make eyes seem wider apart if you tweeze more hairs from the inside corner of each eyebrow.
- If eyes are too wide-set, make them look closer by removing a few hairs from the end of each brow.

Avocado surprise

- If your eyes are puffy, cut thick slices of cold avocado into the shape of two crescents and place one under each eye. Lie down and wait for the swelling to disappear.
- Or use round cucumber slices.

Help for tired eyes

- Relieve the strain of close work by stopping every twenty minutes or so and looking into the distance for sixty seconds. That relaxes the muscles used for focusing.
- Or look out to a faraway object, then back to the close work. Go back and forth a few times.
- And, blink your eyes for a few seconds, close them tightly, blink a few more times, and rest. This lubricates the eyes.
- And, close your eyes for two to three minutes.

Hair's the Question

Don't wash that man right out of your hair

- If you're *really* mad, you may damage your crowning glory. Since hair is at its weakest when it's wet, it's likely to break if you tangle it up by wildly shampooing every which way. Instead, rub gently, following the line of the hair growth.

For better shampooing

- Don't wash hair while you bathe, since soap, residue, dirt, and body chemicals will stay in your hair and make it oily.
- Very hot water will not make hair cleaner and may burn the scalp. Use lukewarm water.
- Don't apply shampoo directly to your head. You'll have a better chance of even coverage if you pour some into your palm, then rub it on.
- Most damage to hair occurs in the drying stage. Don't rough it up with your towel. Instead, pat it dry, then wrap the towel around your head and let it soak up moisture for a few minutes.
- Blow-dry slightly damp hair. If your hair is completely dry, blow-drying may damage it.

Get in condition

- Vinegar rinses became popular when hair was washed with soap. The vinegar would restore natural acids and remove the dull soap film on hair, thus restoring the shine. Since today's shampoos don't contain soap, skip the vinegar and choose a conditioner suitable for your hair type. It'll replace the natural protective oils that coloring and regular shampooing take out.

Two bits' worth of advice

- Too much conditioner will leave your hair dull and without any body. No matter what the label says, mix about a quarter-size dab of conditioner into a cup of hot water. It actually works better than full strength, and it's cheaper.
- The hair nearest the roots gets oils from the scalp. So, start applying your conditioner about two inches from the scalp, using a wide-toothed comb. Be sure to rinse well.

One from column A, two from column B

- Mixing and matching products from different manufacturers isn't a great idea. For example, your shampoo and conditioner may have chemicals that attract one another more than your hair—and wind up locked together, instead of working for you.

Blow-drying like a pro

- Blow-dry hair in the opposite direction from the way you comb it out, and it'll be fuller when it's dry.

Are you splitting hairs?

- Your old brush is likely to have split ends. If you keep using it, so will your hair. Maybe it's time to replace it.

Buying brushes

- Natural bristles are good to use on damaged hair.
- Synthetics are good to use before you shampoo, since they loosen dirt and get hair ready for cleansing.
- A brush with well-spaced, all-natural bristles suits fine, thin hair. Natural bristles won't break or tangle it.
- Medium hair should have some plastic and some natural bristles. Plastic ones make it easier to pull the brush through the hair; natural ones distribute the hair's natural oils.
- For thick, coarse hair, choose a brush with firm, all-plastic bristles.

Cleaning combs

- Soak them in a basin of hot water and a couple of splashes of ammonia. Scrub clean with an old toothbrush.

Natural highlight

- Try mixing the juice of one lemon and two limes together with one ounce of a mild shampoo (it holds the mixture

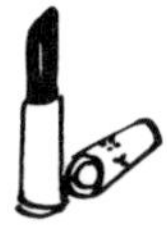

together). Comb it through your *dry* hair with a wide-toothed comb, then sit under the dryer for fifteen to twenty minutes. (Better yet, dry it in the sun.) Then shampoo and condition. If you want to go lighter still, repeat the process a day later.

- Or, wear a frosting cap, pulling hair strands through the weave with a crochet hook. Saturate a cotton ball with the lemon-lime mixture or plain lemon juice and draw it along the strands, then sit in the sun.
- Camomile tea will lighten blond hair. Brew the tea with white wine instead of water to intensify the bleaching, and rinse hair with it over and over. You may need several treatments before you see results.

Using a curling iron on short hair

- Protect your scalp by slipping a comb into hair roots.

To condition or revitalize?

- Confused between revitalizers and conditioners? Conditioners are meant to be rinsed off, while revitalizers are applied and left on. You need a revitalizer occasionally if you blow-dry, brush or tease your hair, color it, or are outdoors a lot.

Down with the frizzies

- Frizzy hair may be more manageable if you try setting it first, then blow-drying.

For dry, crackly hair

- If your hair stands on end even when you're not at a horror movie, try using a brush and comb with fewer, smoother bristles, preferably of wood or metal. They move through the hair faster and cause less static.
- If hair still crackles, try rubbing a little conditioner on your hands, then smoothing them over your hair.

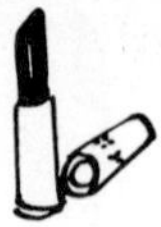

- Or spray hair spray or the static-free product used for clothing on your brush before styling.
- Or, lightly rub a fabric-softener sheet over hair.

Hair-spray hint

- Your spray can won't clog if you hold it upside down after each use and spray until it stops. That empties the nozzle.

In the swim

- If your hair keeps turning green after a swim in the pool, ask your hairdresser about the new swimmers' shampoos on the market. There are versions for both colored and uncolored hair.

Roots showing? Try the magic wand

- Your mascara wand can be used to do an emergency touch-up job on dark hair if you're overdue at the hairdresser's. For light hair, shake on some talcum and brush lightly.

Hair today, gone tomorrow

- Did you know that having sexual relations, or even anticipating them, can make your hair grow faster? (This is a benefit of baldness: No one has a clue about your private life.)
- Certain medications, megadoses of vitamin A, high fever, lack of protein, and seasonal shedding (it peaks in autumn in the Northern Hemisphere) are all causes of hair loss.

Keep your equipment in shape

- Hair dryers need an occasional cleaning. Use your vacuum cleaner and run the brush attachment over the blower end.
- Electric rollers should be washed occasionally in shampoo

and warm water, and scrubbed with an old toothbrush. Otherwise they'll get your hair dirty.

If you overdo the dye

- Flashing a new color that's as subtle as a fire gong? Don't panic. Buy a "temporary drabbing rinse" in an ash-colored shade.

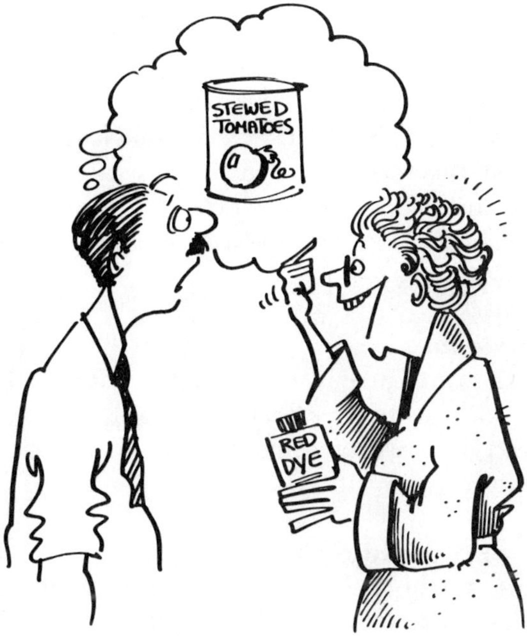

- Is the skin around your hairline stained from your tint? Simply rub leftover tint into the stained area and rinse with water.

Don't dye the sink

- Before putting henna or color on your hair, coat the sink lightly with liquid dishwashing detergent. The sink won't stain from the dye.

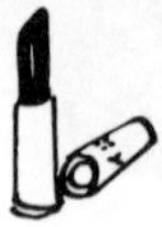

Toothy Matters

Paste for healthy gums

- Contrary to popular belief, the biggest cause of tooth loss in adults is not tooth decay but gum disease. Try to avoid it by daily applications of a paste made of baking soda moistened with hydrogen peroxide. Smear the paste along the gums at the tooth line, massage with a rubber tip or toothpick, and then with an electric toothbrush. Finish up with a salt solution delivered by Water Pik, and floss thoroughly.

Toothpicks vs. floss

- Toothpicks aren't nearly as effective as dental floss for removing food particles. Besides, toothpicks can scratch enamel and harm your gums. Save them for spearing hors d'oeuvres.

Caring for your toothbrush

- Keep your toothbrush hung so it will air-dry and water won't collect at the base of the bristles.
- Dentists recommend replacing toothbrushes every two months. Bent, worn bristles don't do a good job of cleaning.

When to floss

- Floss *before* brushing with fluoride toothpaste. Then the side surfaces are clean, so fluoride comes in direct contact with the enamel.

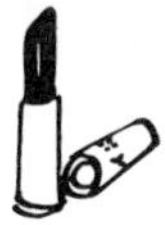

Checking your toothbrush technique

- Buy a three-week supply of "disclosing tablets" from the drugstore. They temporarily stain any plaque a dark pink color and you have to brush to remove it. You'll soon learn which areas you tend to neglect.

Don't stockpile toothpaste

- Fluoride loses its cavity-fighting effectiveness after about six months on the shelf. This is one case where you shouldn't load up on a bargain. Instead, buy fresh toothpaste as needed.

You'll wonder where the enamel went

- Tooth whiteners scrub away some tooth stains, but they also remove enamel—which doesn't grow back. Avoid them in favor of regular professional dental cleanings.

Don't forget to brush your tongue

- Food can accumulate in the irregular surfaces and decay, causing an extreme case of bad breath. This is easily corrected if you also brush your tongue when you brush your teeth.

It's a wash

- The FDA found that *none* of thirty-four ingredients used in mouthwashes was safe and effective, and ten shouldn't be used at all.

Sugared cereals

- The American Dental Association tests many separate foods in a single category to find out which produce the most cavities. Whether they have 6 percent, 15 percent, or 60 percent sugar, sugared breakfast cereals have almost equal decay-producing potential.

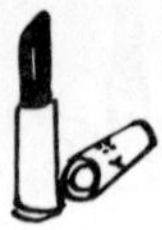

Say "cheese"

- Cheddar cheese may slow tooth decay. It did with laboratory rats who were fed the cheese directly after eating sugar, a known contributor to tooth decay. The cheese may interfere with the action of bacteria that produce a certain acid which causes tooth decay.

Take your dentures to the dentist

- As many as 70 percent of denture wearers haven't visited the dentist in five years, but that's bad health practice. Dentures should be checked to see whether the jaw or bone is being harmed.

Bite down

- Denture wearers should try to chew with equal weight on both sides to cut bone loss and avoid excessive wear on one side.

Clenching your teeth?

- Teeth clenchers may have "tense jaw syndrome." Get relief with this exercise: Drop your jaw open, moving it back and forth to a comfortable position. Gently massage jaw muscles, then close your eyes and relax in that position for a minute.

Acupressure for a toothache

- If the toothache's on the left, press together the thumb and forefinger of the left hand. If toothache's on the right, use the right hand. See the bump the muscle forms? Relax your hand and massage the spot on the hand where the bump was, using ice wrapped in gauze, for seven minutes. You should be pain-free for up to a half hour. Repeat as needed. Works better than a cold pack on the cheek.

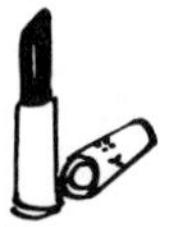

Saving a tooth

- If someone in the family loses a tooth, rinse it in water (don't scrub) and pop it back in. Then get to the dentist, who'll put in a splint to help it reimplant itself.
- Or, drop it into a cup of milk to carry to the dentist for reimplanting.
- Or, wrap carefully in a wet piece of gauze and hold it under your tongue en route to the dentist.

Temporary caps and fillings

- If you should lose a cap or filling and a dentist isn't available, don't panic: you can make yourself a temporary replacement. All you need is two drugstore items: zinc oxide and oil of cloves (eugenol). They mix together to form a white paste that hardens quickly. Just pack the paste into the cavity, clean up the edges, and it will last for two or three days until you can get to a dentist.

Preventing canker sores

- Avoid eating sharp food like peanut brittle, use a medium or soft-bristled toothbrush. Physical damage to the lining of the mouth starts most canker sores.

Show of Hands

Condition while you work

- Two in one: Apply conditioner such as hand lotion before slipping on rubber gloves and let the heat of dishwashing help the cream sink in.

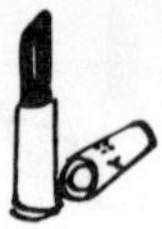

- Or, in winter, apply conditioner, slip on cotton gloves, and then slip your hands into heavier gloves. Hands will be thoroughly moisturized by the time you unpeel.

If you wear rubber gloves

- You may get chapping under rubber gloves when moisture is trapped inside. Avoid this by buying gloves a size too large, then wearing a pair of cotton gloves beneath them.

Handy hint

- Expensive hand lotions are no improvement over pure glycerin (available at drugstores). Apply it at night before retiring and almost overnight your hands will look 100 percent better.
- To get the most benefit from glycerin or any other lotion, first soak your hands in warm water before applying. Warm water opens the pores and the lotion is absorbed better.

Get the red out

- A rub of fresh lemon helps bleach out redness on hands.

Cause for applause

- If your hands are cold or tired, massage them. Stroke from tip of finger toward palm, spending about five minutes on each hand.

Super glue remover

- Don't try to peel dried glue off your skin. Instead, soak the glue-covered area in nail-polish remover until the glue disappears.

Wedding ring making you itchy?

- That redness, irritation, and itch under your wedding band and other rings may be caused by built-up soap trapped

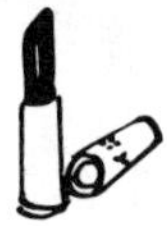

underneath. Slide the ring off, rinse your hands thoroughly, and apply a hydrocortisone cream.

- Or, boil your ring in soapy water, and don't wear it for two or three days until the itch disappears.
- Or, pierce a vitamin E capsule and apply the fluid generously several times a day until itch has gone away.

At Your Fingertips

Making nails grow

- Drinking unflavored gelatin is now considered to be of no help in making nails grow. Although nails are made of protein, taking in extra protein (in gelatin or any other form) has no effect on their growth, and a Columbia Uni-

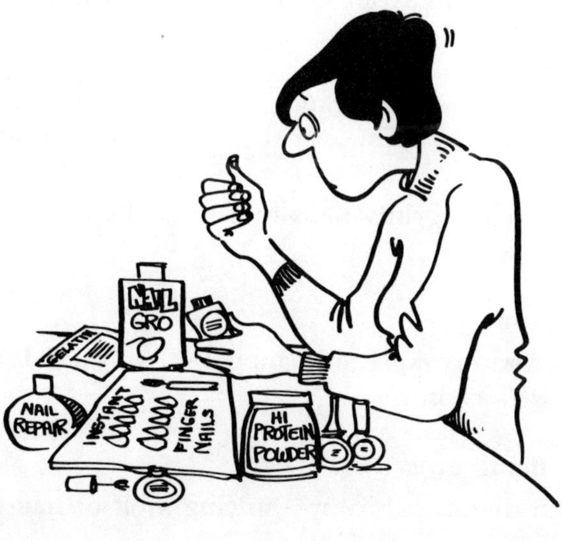

versity nutritionist adds that gelatin in particular is lacking in a necessary nutrient for nail growth.

- However, typing does help nails grow slightly faster. So do playing the piano, summer weather, and pregnancy.
- Or try tapping your finger on a hard surface or massaging the base of your nails. This stimulates the half-moon section, and helps develop stronger, thicker nails.

For extra protection

- If you're doing household jobs, take special care of nails by putting a strip of masking tape over each one before you slip on the gloves.
- Try to use nail-polish remover no more than once a week. More frequent use can dry out your nails and cause them to split.

Keeping the dirt out

- Scrape your nails over a bar of soap before you work in the garden. Dirt won't collect underneath. Also, wear gloves when possible to avoid scratches and bruises.

Gentle on your hands

- If you want a gentler cleaning than you'd get from a brush, work cleansing cream over the surface of nails and under the tips.
- Or soak really grimy nails in a mild shampoo and water solution.

A tip for you

- You'll avoid breaking and chipping if you polish *under* nail tips as well as on top.

Between manicures

- You can mend a chip by applying a bit of nail-polish re-

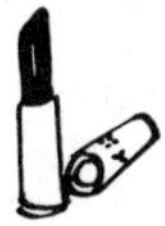

mover with a cotton swab, smoothing the edges of the area. When it's dry, apply a fresh coat of polish.

- If you've chipped off some nail as well as some polish, smooth off the rough edges with an emery board before you fill in more polish.
- If polish has worn off just at nail tip, apply a thin coat along edges only, then blend the whole thing by applying a top coat.

To break in an emery board

- A new file is often too coarse and rough for your nails. Before using it, rub the coarse side over another emery board for a few seconds.

Techniques for filing and buffing

- Don't "saw" with an emery board. Use long, sweeping strokes.
- Buff from cuticle to tip. A back-and-forth motion causes heat to build up. That can damage nails.
- If you hold your nail file at a slight angle, each layer of nail will be slightly longer than the one underneath. This helps prevent splitting.
- For longer, stronger fingernails, make sure that when you file you leave sides straight, rounding the nails at the tips only. Snags occur at the sides of nails.

Special problems

- Sometimes a person's nails are in bad shape because of an allergy to food or cosmetics. Consult your doctor if you suspect that may be the case.
- Ridges the length of your nail may indicate a lack of vitamin A.
- White spots can be caused by a blow but may also reveal illness, zinc deficiency, a nervous problem, or extreme cold.

- Thin, splitting or pitted nails may show you need calcium, protein, or sulfur.
- Brittle nails may indicate general ill health or lack of vitamin C, protein, or folic acid.
- Cracking may mean vitamin deficiency—especially vitamin B_3.
- Opaque bands on your fingertips may indicate poor protein reserve, and/or shortage of vitamin A.
- Loose nails? You may need iron.

Hot oil treatments

- Lubricating hot oil treatments, formerly available only in salons, are now sold in kit form in drugstores. They help condition nails and cuticles.

Nail sculpture and wraps

- The plastic paste used to "sculpt" a new nail may cause allergic reactions like pain, bleeding, or infection, possibly even loss of a nail. The new nail might even be deformed because of the injury.
- Nail wrapping—thin paper strips applied to nail and coated with glue—may cause similar problems if you're allergic to the glue.
- Fake tips are a little less risky because the glue generally covers only the nail's edge.
- Safest nail wrap involves coating nail with a liquid containing nylon fibers. The coating is applied first in one direction, then in another to form a strong grid pattern.

Caring for your cuticles

- Don't cut cuticles. They are nature's way of keeping dirt and bacteria out of the nail base area.

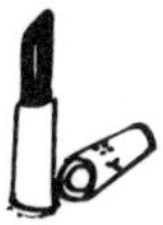

- Use a wooden orange stick, not a metal tool, to avoid damage.
- If you use cuticle-remover solution, follow instructions on the bottle carefully. If left on too long, the solution can cause burns and other irritations.
- Salty or chlorinated water can be hard on cuticles. So, before swimming coat them with a dab of petroleum jelly.
- To clean cuticles, insert fingertips in half a lemon and wiggle them around.

To remove stains from fingertips

- The tips of your nails are very porous and may be stained by cigarettes, food, cosmetics, etc. Bleach stains away with a lemon half! Wiggle your fingertips in it, then rinse with lukewarm water.

Get set

- Oops! Just finished your manicure and already you've smudged it? Take the polish brush, dip it into a capful of polish remover, and brush it over the smudge once or twice.
- Polish usually takes thirty minutes to set. But dipping a fresh manicure into very cold water helps it set quicker.

Hangnails your hangup?

- Get a cream containing 10 percent urea from the drugstore. Massage it into the afflicted area several times a day. You should see an improvement in two or three days.

Cure for nail biters

- Try the same trick moms use to stop kids from sucking thumbs: a little of that bitter liquid swabbed on your hands. The taste will remind you to stop biting. It's available in drugstores.

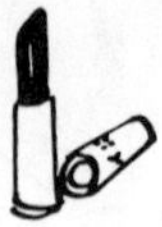

Getting Soaked

A fragrant soak to soothe you

- Tie a spoonful each of dried lavender flowers, rosemary, thyme, and dried mint in a double thickness of cheesecloth. Put it into the tub, pour very hot water over the bag, and let it steep for ten minutes. Then finish filling the tub and soak away!

For a more comfortable soak

- The ideal temperature for bathwater is between 96 and 98 degrees F.—the same as body temperature.

Bath nourishment for your skin

- Mix a half cup of corn oil into one quart of whole milk and pour into the bath.
- Or, instead of the whole milk, mix a cup of powdered skim milk with three cups of lukewarm water, then add to bath. Or pour the powdered milk into a handkerchief or double cheesecloth bag and swish the bag around in your bathwater.

Bubble trouble

- It's hard to believe that there can be a problem with something as wonderful as bubble bath, but it can remove the skin's natural oil. This can cause drying, fissuring, and irritation, and even lead to infection. The danger's greater if you soak long and often. So, like good food and good wine, enjoy in moderation!

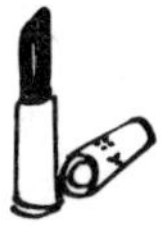

Bath soaps by skin type

- If your skin is dry, select superfatted soaps containing cold cream, coconut oil, lanolin, or even cocoa butter.
- Oily skin reacts better to non-fatted glycerin or "soapless" types.
- Try a bland soap if your problem is blemished or sensitive skin. Medicated soaps should be used only if recommended by a doctor.

Hard-water solution

- Glycerin soap lathers easier and cleans better than other soaps in hard water.

Hang that loofah high

- Loofahs can get moldy if they don't dry between uses. If yours doesn't have a loop attached, cut a hole and thread a cord through it for hanging.

Salt-water bath?

- Half a cup of table salt in the bathwater helps guard against vaginal infections.

Hot oatmeal bath

- This helps cure itchy skin problems. Pour some oatmeal in cheesecloth, tie shut, and hang from the spigot so bathwater runs through it—or use the pouch as a sponge while you bathe.
- You can also use oatmeal on any rough spots. Make a paste of the instant type mixed with water and apply to knees, elbows, feet. Let it set awhile, then rub off with washcloth.

Bath oil

- Add bath oil to the tub only after you've soaked ten minutes, or the oil will act as a barrier between your skin and the water.

Best time to moisturize

- Apply moisturizer immediately after getting out of bath or shower to trap moisture in the skin.

Footnotes

What amazing "feats"

- You'll walk 65,000 miles—2½ times around the globe—in your lifetime, even if you never leave home.
- You put 1,000 tons of pressure on your feet each day.
- A one-mile run puts 200 tons of stress on each foot of a 125-pound runner.
- A fourth of all the bones of your body are in your feet: fifty-two in all.
- Housework takes you on an 8½-mile walk each day.
- Considering all the hard work our feet do, it's no wonder four out of five Americans have some foot abnormality.

And the last shall be first

- The parts of your body you probably think the least about—your feet—actually have two nice things going for them: they don't always get fat when the rest of you does, and they are the least vulnerable to signs of aging.

If your back aches, blame your feet

- Eighty percent of the population has foot abnormalities, and about the same number have back problems. Minor foot problems such as a callus or corn and poor weight distribution can affect your walk and eventually your back. Maybe your podiatrist can help.

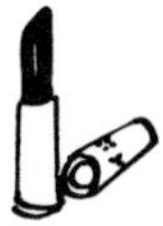

Barefootin'

- Exercise and air your feet by walking barefoot on soft surfaces, such as carpeting and grass. Avoid walking barefoot on wet public areas such as the concrete around swimming pools—these places can incubate viral growths, such as plantar warts.

Feet killing you?

- Take off those spike heels. Podiatrists recommend ½″ to 1¾″ as maximum heel height. They also recommend switching between low and medium heels.
- Try foam insoles for shock absorption. Those containing nitrogen wear better than others.

If the shoe fits

- When you try on shoes, remember that heels shouldn't slip. Boot heels, however, should slip just a little bit.
- Shoes should be a quarter to half an inch longer than your big toe, and shouldn't gap when you stand on tiptoe.
- Arches should be rigid but soles should be soft enough to cushion feet (crepe, rubber, or flexible leather soles are best).
- Shop at night. Your feet swell as much as half a size between morning and evening.
- Try on both left and right shoes. If one of your feet is larger than the other, you may have an uncomfortable fit in certain styles.
- Back of the shoe around the heel shouldn't sag and should be reinforced, preferably with leather.
- Correctly fitting shoes can prevent 99 percent of all foot complaints.

On your toes

Here are some ways to relax your feet:

- Roll a rolling pin, tennis ball, small bottle, or even a can of beer under your bare feet for a few minutes every day.
- Lie down, placing your feet against a hard surface. "Walk" your feet up the surface, grasping with wide-spread toes.

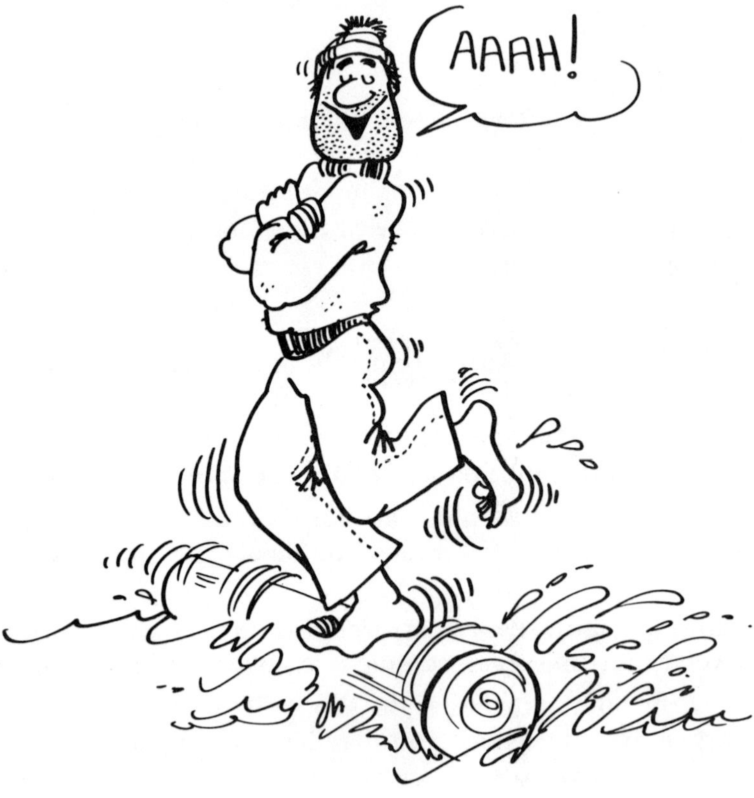

- Try to put your feet up as often as possible.

Sole food

- To make tired feet feel good, soak them for ten minutes in warm water steeped with mint leaves or tea bags.

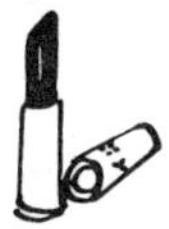

- Or soak them in a basin of warm water to which you've added a fourth of a cup each of salt and baking soda.
- Soften them with warmed vegetable oil, then wrap in a damp hot towel and sit for ten minutes.
- After soaking, rub calluses with a rough towel, massage in two tablespoons oil and a teaspoon of vinegar.
- Follow a pumice-stone rub with a thin coating of white vegetable cooking shortening.
- Some people swear that frequent applications of castor oil will make corns or calluses disappear.

A smooth idea

- Apply glycerin before using pumice stone. The combination is better than using either moisturizer or pumice alone.

Caring for pumice

- If it gets too soft, buff it up by rubbing it across sandpaper or concrete.

Hot foot, or cold feet?

- To revive and refresh hot, tired feet quickly, put them under the faucet and blast them with cold water. It stimulates circulation and loosens up your muscles. In fact, because of all the nerve endings in your feet, you'll feel better all over.
- If your feet have been out in the cold, help them recover by soaking in warm water to which you've added a cup of Epsom salts.

Powder perfect

- To avoid irritation and blisters, use baby or foot powder to absorb moisture. Sprinkle it all over your feet, but especially between your toes. Also dust the insides of your shoes.

- Cornstarch is good to use if your feet are blistered.

Sock it to you

- Choose wool or cotton socks. They absorb perspiration more effectively than synthetics do.
- Wear two pairs of socks (a thicker one over a thinner pair) to reduce chances of blistering when playing tennis or other sports.

Athlete's foot

- Since warmth and moisture create the best environment for athlete's foot, make sure socks are washed after each wearing.
- Allow shoes to dry thoroughly between wearings.
- Avoid deodorant soaps, since they remove surface-protecting oils and tend to irritate the skin.
- Cornstarch helps avoid dampness and reduces friction.
- You'll perspire less if you drink less caffeine-containing beverages such as coffee, tea, and cola.

Washing shoes

- Since your feet sweat about one glass of water a day, washable canvas sneakers (ideally, ones with terry linings) are best. Because they don't "breathe," non-washable canvas and vinyl styles help promote fungus growth.

Removing leg hair

- Always shave after a bath, rather than before. Leg hairs plump up with water and are easier to get off.
- Shaving against the grain gets closer results. But if you get ingrown hairs, shave down.

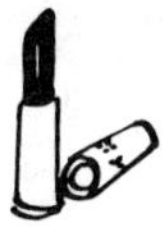

- The hair on the upper thigh shouldn't be shaved. Instead, remove it with a depilatory or wax, or bleach it.
- If you use a depilatory, the speediest way to clean up afterward is to get into a shower.

Chapter 5

Here's to Living Well
HEALTH

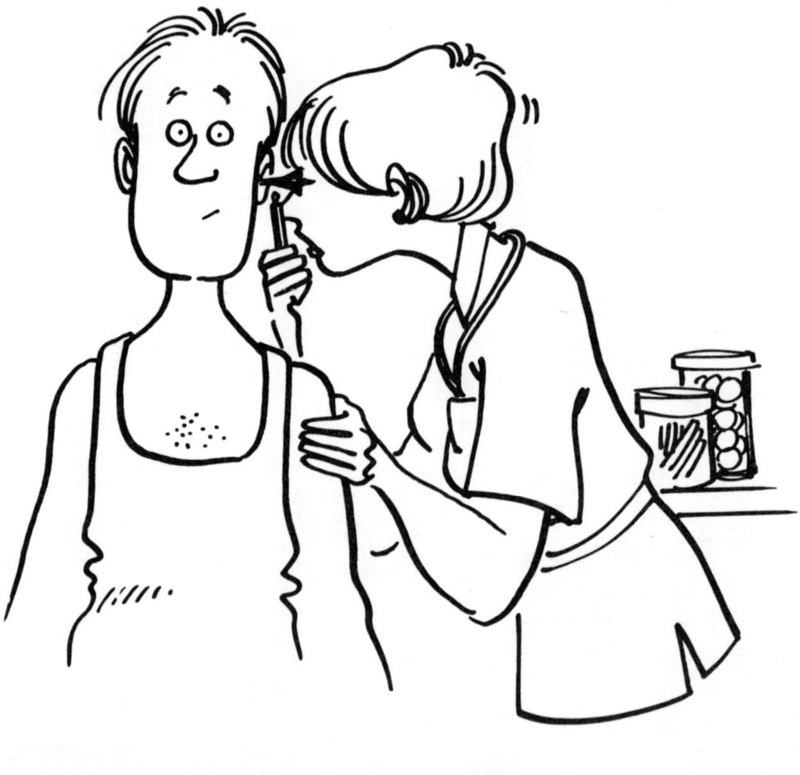

Relieving Stress

All wound up

- If you're tired and irritable, can't sleep, having stomach or breathing problems, stress may be the problem. Even pleasant changes—buying a new house, becoming pregnant, getting married—can cause the same stress symptoms as calamities. Many people find that exercise is the best method for calming down (and it also tones you up).

Breathe to relax

- Breathing from the diaphragm instead of the chest can relax you and help relieve stress. Here's how. Lie on the floor, arms at sides, or sit straight, hands on thighs. Go limp and breathe normally. When the breathing is rhythmic, make each exhale twice as long as an inhale. (If you put a hand at the lower edge of the rib cage, you can feel the air coming into the diaphragm.) Repeat for five to ten minutes, open eyes slowly, and rest a minute or so before getting up.

Stomach "in knots"

- Studies have shown that stress slows down food digestion, so there's some truth to the saying about a stomach being "all tied up in knots." If that's how yours feels at the end of a hectic day, take ten to fifteen minutes just before a meal to sip a glass of water slowly . . . and *relax.*

That lump in your throat

- It could be a response to stress. Try breathing slowly and deeply so the muscles that cause that sensation will unclench and relax.

Fishing for a stress reliever?

- Consider buying an aquarium (why do you think all those doctors have them in their offices?). Gazing into one can actually reduce blood pressure. It's better than watching television!

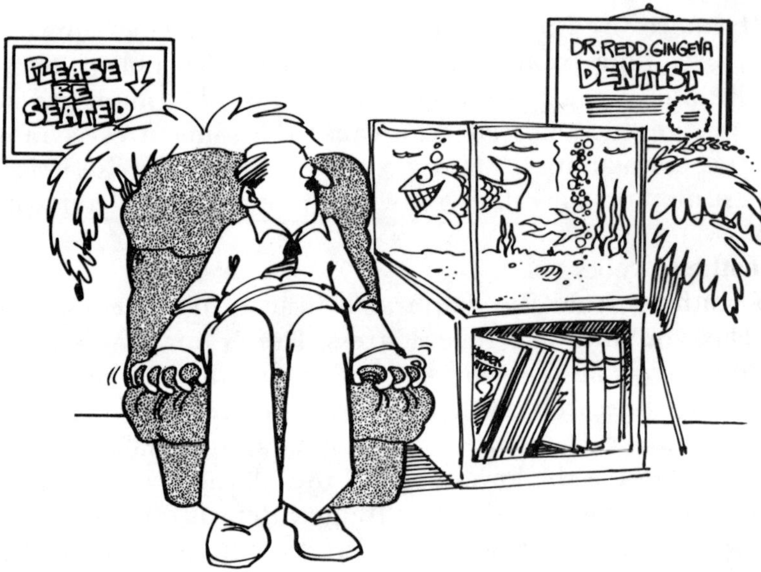

What to eat in times of stress

- Don't turn to pacifiers like sweets. If you're having a rough time, your body loses its reserves of vitamins A and C faster than normally, so eat foods packed with these nutrients: dark green and yellow vegetables for A; citrus fruits, baked potato, strawberries, green peppers for C. Also take in proteins, especially milk products, which contain riboflavin and calcium.

Coloring your behavior

- Researchers think that different colors can cause different behavior reactions in yourself and others. For example, certain shades of pink may act as a sedative and possibly even relax muscles. The brain reacts to pink by slowing the release of adrenaline into your system, which in turn slows the heart muscle and calms you down. So if you're planning to ask your boss for a raise, wear pink.

Visiting the Doctor

Selecting a physician

- If you're seeking a new family physician, write to the American Academy of Family Physicians, 1740 E. 92nd St., Kansas City, MO 64114, for their directory.
- If you want to find out about any doctor's training and qualifications, check your library to see if they have the *Directory of Medical Specialists.*

Time for a checkup?

- The American Medical Association suggests that healthy adults over twenty-one should see the doctor at five-year intervals, and after forty every one to three years—unless you've got a special cause for concern.

What's up, doc?

- If it's your blood pressure, your M.D. may be the cause! Twenty percent of patients in one study who had mild hypertension during a checkup had normal pressure at home. The anxiety of the office visit sent it up.

Less waiting time

- You're less likely to be sitting around the waiting room with rising blood pressure if you choose appointments at these times:

Lunch hours (all doctors)
Tuesdays or Thursdays for general practitioners
December for dentists
Midwinter or early spring for eye doctors
Evenings for pharmacists
Midsummer and Friday afternoons for gynecologists

Making a checkup count

- Tell the doctor what your *symptoms* are—not what you *think* your illness is.
- Give the doctor specific details about any past medical problems.
- Tell the doctor exactly how you feel without waiting for him to "discover" a problem.
- See if you can be specific. For example, a pain may be dull, sharp, throbbing, squeezing.

Questions your doctor should answer

- What is my problem?
- What caused it?
- What should I do about it? (And write down the answers.)
- What should I do if I don't get better?
- Should I return to you, and when?

A breath test to gauge your health

- Low results on a forced vital capacity (FVC) breath test may indicate that you are at risk for heart attack, stroke, or other cardiovascular or respiratory diseases. At your next physical, you might ask your doctor if he recommends the test—so you can take precautionary measures.

Two opinions are better than one

- In non-emergency cases such as hernia repair and tonsillectomies, see a second doctor. Thirty-one percent of the time, they don't advise an operation. Your insurance company will probably pay for the second visit.
- Call Second-Opinion Hotline toll free 1-800-638-6833 if you need the name of another doctor.

Shortening a hospital stay

- Ask your doctor whether you can get preoperative tests as an outpatient. You may save a day or two in the hospital.
- If you have a choice, don't check in on a weekend. Most non-emergency surgeries are performed between Monday morning and Friday afternoon.

Taking Your Medicine

Deciphering the prescription

- You might be interested to know some of the most common instructions on the prescriptions doctors write:
  a.c.—before meals
  ad—up to
  ad lib—as required
  b.i.d.—twice daily
  c̄ (line over c)—with
  gtt—drops
  h.s.—at bedtime
  p.c.—after meals
  p.r.n.—as needed
  q.i.d.—four times daily
  qh—hourly

q4h—every four hours
sig—label
s̄ (line over s)—without
stat—immediately
t.i.d.—three times a day
ut dict.—as directed

Are you overdosing?

- It's been estimated that three or four billion of the ten billion dollars Americans spend each year on non-prescription drugs are wasted on products that are overpriced, unsafe, or ineffective.

Tough pill to swallow

- It's not as simple as you thought! The American Medical Association says to swallow a tablet by placing it on the tongue, sipping water and tilting your head back. But with a capsule, tilt head forward while swallowing. The capsule weighs less than water, so the forward motion will flush it down your throat.

To get medicine down, stand up

- If you take medication while you're lying down, you may delay its entry into your bloodstream and cause yourself nausea and heartburn if it remains in your esophagus. Unless you're confined to bed, stand up to swallow and remain standing for ninety seconds.
- And always take tablets or capsules with at least a full glass of fluid. This is especially important with aspirin, to minimize stomach irritation. (It also helps to take aspirin immediately after a meal.)

Aspirin by any other name

- *All* aspirin products contain only one ingredient proved safe and effective: aspirin. Don't spend from two to five times as much for the brand-name products. Buy generic aspirin.

- In most cases, you don't need "extra-strength" tablets. One or two generic aspirins are equivalent, so don't waste your money on expensive extra-strength brands.

Capsule or tablet?

- Buy the tablet form of a drug if possible. Capsules generally cost more and produce just about the same effect.

Take C, not tea

- If you're taking an iron supplement, don't take it together with your tea. The tannic acid in tea can block the absorption of iron and even, in extreme cases, lead to anemia. If you take it with a vitamin C-rich food (such as orange or tomato juice), the vitamin C will help the iron absorption.

Taking water pills?

- If you take any diuretic to relieve excessive fluids, you may be losing potassium, which results in muscle cramps, weakness, faster heart rate. Make up for the loss by eating potassium-rich foods such as citrus fruits, bananas, baked potatoes.

Rubbing alcohol

- Use it only for minor skin irritations (insect bites, for example). On open wounds, it may actually cause infection.

A checkup for your medicine chest

- These preparations can keep indefinitely in a cool, dry place: petroleum jelly, Mercurochrome, Merthiolate, bicarbonate of soda, mineral oil, boric acid, rubbing alcohol. But check all other items, prescription and non-prescription, to see whether they have expired. If in doubt, call your pharmacist.

Water Log

Different kinds of water

- Distilled is the purest. Great for steam irons, but tastes flat.
- Still water is just uncarbonated water (with no carbon dioxide), like tap water.
- Sparkling water is naturally effervescent or tap water with carbon dioxide added.
- Mineral water is usually tap water with added minerals such as magnesium, potassium, calcium, and sodium. But "natural mineral water" comes from a source in which minerals are naturally dissolved.
- Spring water comes from a spring, but may be processed. (Carbonation may have been added.)
- Seltzer is tap water that's been filtered, with carbon dioxide added.
- Club soda is seltzer plus minerals and mineral salts.

What's mixed in the mixer?

- Soda waters such as seltzer, club soda, and natural sparkling water are regulated by the same standards as ordinary soft drinks such as cola. They may contain up to .05 percent alcohol and .02 percent caffeine. Check the labels before you buy.

Low-sodium diets and water

- Avoid club soda. It can be high in sodium. Choose seltzer instead; it has no added salts.
- Even sparkling waters can have a high sodium content. The lower ones are Perrier, Evian, and Mountain Valley, while

Saratoga, Vichy Celestins, and San Pellegrino are relatively high in sodium. Read the labels.

- Some water systems have more than eight times the recommended amount of sodium, which is 20 mg. per liter. Your local health department or water company can tell you about your drinking water. If it's too high in sodium, you might consider switching to a bottled water or a water-purifying system.

Make a homemade purifier
- Put a coffee filter in a large funnel.
- Wash enough granular activated carbon to fill one fourth of the funnel. (To wash carbon, put in a jar, fill with water, cover and shake. After the carbon settles, pour off the water at the top. Repeat until the water you pour off is clear.)
- Set the funnel in a large jar, add washed carbon, and slowly pour tap water through funnel.
- Change carbon every three weeks or after twenty gallons of water have been filtered through it.
- Store filtered water, covered, in refrigerator.

Water for the camper
- No matter how clean that mountain stream or babbling brook might look, don't drink from it unless you're sure it's safe. Even purifying tablets don't kill certain parasites that cause diarrhea. It's best to be cautious: strain the water, then boil it for ten minutes.

An alternative to boiling water
- To purify untested or cloudy water, use liquid chlorine laundry bleach. Add two drops per quart of clear water, or four drops per quart of cloudy. Mix thoroughly, let stand for twenty minutes. If you can't detect a slight

chlorine odor, repeat, letting the water stand for fifteen minutes more.

Your Aching Head

Does being a woman give you a headache?

- If misery does love company, it might ease your pain to know that 85 percent of the 45 million headache sufferers in America are women.

Ten kinds of headaches you may never have known you had

- Chinese restaurant syndrome: comes from too much monosodium glutamate in your food—Chinese or other kinds.
- Hot dog headache: from nitrates or nitrites added to hot dogs, ham, bacon. If you boil these meats, the additives dissolve.
- Ice-cream headache: from sudden cooling of the roof of the mouth, which affects the nerves. Sip cold foods slowly.
- Caffeine withdrawal: If you're used to caffeine, blood vessels are constricted. Take it away, and they dilate. Withdraw slowly to avoid a headache.
- Hunger: from not eating enough, or from eating too much. Excess sweets may cause your pancreas to create a lot of insulin, and your blood sugar becomes too low. Snack on high-protein foods instead (nuts, fruits, vegetables).
- Noxious fumes headaches: from crowded highways; also from formaldehyde, found in plywood and home insulating materials.

- Bruxism headache: from grinding your teeth at night, or from excessive gum chewing.
- Turtle headache: If you sleep with the covers over your head, you build up carbon dioxide (or you can get it from a crowded room). Tuck covers in so you can't pull them up. Or if you're doing it to avoid light, try wearing a sleep mask.
- Sunstroke headache: Body is dehydrated from the sun, so drink small amounts of warm water over a two- or three-hour period.
- Salt: Stay away from highly salted snack foods.

News giving you a headache?

- It may be the newsprint! People who suspect they may be allergic to newsprint and other chemicals common in our environment, such as aerosols, scouring powders, etc., can get information from the Society of Clinical Ecology, 2005 Franklin St., Suite 490, Denver, CO 80205. (Enclose a self-addressed stamped envelope.)

Diet for migraine

- Migraine sufferers may be allergic to foods—especially wheat, milk, rice, eggs, fish, chocolate, tomatoes, oranges, cheese, tea, or coffee. If you get migraines, your doctor may want you to try eliminating some of these foods from your diet.
- Some migraine victims get relief from eating frequently, or staying on a high-protein, low-carbohydrate diet.

Hot and cold for headaches

- When a headache starts, try pressing alternately hot and cold compresses to the back of your head and neck for ten minutes.
- Or drink ice water or suck on ice cubes.

A bright thought for your headache

- Tension headaches sometimes can be caused by eyestrain from working under poor lighting conditions. Maybe a new lamp would help.

Just the (Cold) Facts

Before you visit the doctor

- You might want to bear in mind that ten to twenty percent of doctor visits are made by people with simple upper respiratory infections (colds)—for which he can do nothing.

Did you know . . .

- Consumers spend well over $1.5 billion dollars a year on non-prescription drugs to relieve colds, allergies, and asthma.
- Advertisers spend $150 million persuading them to do it.

Common misconceptions about the common cold

- That your sore throat is a strep throat. Strep is usually a children's disease. In adults, sore throat is just another cold symptom.
- That your coughing means bronchitis. The chances are it's not, unless you're high-risk, like a middle-aged smoker with damaged lungs.
- That there's a cure. Even though your doctor may prescribe antibiotics, there is no cure for the common cold.

Button up your overcoat—and stay away from me!

- No matter what Mom told you, colds don't come automatically from sitting in drafts, not dressing warmly, or going out with wet hair (although when any of these lowers your body temperature, germs may more successfully attack). You get most colds in winter because you're inside, and poor air circulation helps transmission of viruses.

Money savers for colds

- The cheapest, best way to treat a cold is just to let it take its course.
- But if you want to relieve a particular symptom, don't buy the more expensive preparations designed to relieve several problems. Buy a specific one (see list below).
- Buy generic products when possible.

Which ingredient does what

- An antihistamine relieves sneezing and watery, itchy eyes.
- A nasal decongestant will open clogged nasal passages. Look for drops and sprays with oxymetazoline hydrochloride, xylometazoline hydrochloride, or phenylephrine hydrochloride.
- Antitussives suppress coughs. If a cough prevents you from sleeping, try a product with dextromethorphan.
- Expectorants will loosen mucus to be coughed up.
- A bronchodilator will enlarge bronchial passages, make it easier for an asthma sufferer to breathe.
- Anticholinergics dry up watery secretions in the nose and eyes.

Let it run

- If you can stand it, a runny nose is best left untreated. It helps promote draining, which allows your body to get rid of the virus.

Rules for blowing your nose (even if you thought it came naturally)

- *Do* blow gently and often. You'll clear the mucus out.
- *Don't* stop up one nostril and blow through the other. You may force mucus up the Eustachian tubes and cause an ear infection.

A cold remedy out of your fridge

- Squeeze a lemon, add eight ounces of water, and sweeten with honey. Then add ice and sip through a straw. Or, if you're congested, drink it hot.

Hot foods for colds

- Mother was right: take chicken soup when you've got a cold—or any hot liquid. Researchers have found that hot liquids increase mucus flow, which helps end the infection more quickly.
- Or try something really hot. Eat horseradish, chili, mustard, pepper, or gargle with ten to twenty drops of Tabasco sauce in a glass of water. Hot foods help clear out the respiratory tract.

Keeping colds away

- Washing your hands often may keep you free of sniffles, since colds may be contracted by touching the skin of an infected person. So keep your hands clean and avoid rubbing your eyes and nose.

Christmas and the common cold

- Christmas and New Year's are traditional peak times for catching cold, because you're in crowded rooms with poor circulation and because you're under stress, which helps increase your susceptibility. Try to get as much rest as possible.

- It's also possible, if you get an annual "cold" around the holidays (runny nose, itchy eyes, hoarseness), that you may be allergic to your Christmas tree like four million others. To test, stow your tree outdoors for a couple of days. If the "cold" disappears, go for the fabulous fake next year.

Feed a cold, feed a fever

- Since *any* infection causes your body to burn extra calories, the medical community now suggests that you eat and drink more both when you're sniffling and when you're shivering. If you don't feel like eating, get your calories from fruit juice.

Hot tips for fever

- It's okay to bathe or shower in lukewarm water. As moisture evaporates, your temperature may even drop.
- Sponge with tepid water rather than alcohol. (There have been problems with alcohol inhalation in a poorly ventilated room.)
- Don't keep the blankets piled on. Let excess body heat escape or temperature won't drop, and may even climb.
- Call a doctor when the temperature is above 104 degrees for an adult or 105 degrees for a child, when it continues for more than twenty-four hours without cause or more than seventy-two hours no matter what the cause; or when a child under three months has any temperature.

Is the thermometer accurate?

- If the mercury won't easily shake down to normal or won't hold long enough to read, you need a new thermometer.

An accurate temperature

- Put the thermometer way back under the tongue. That's where the heat pockets are that best reflect your temperature.

Let me feel your forehead

- Don't just touch hands to the forehead of someone who may have a temperature. Touch both your hands *and* your face, then touch a well person for comparison.

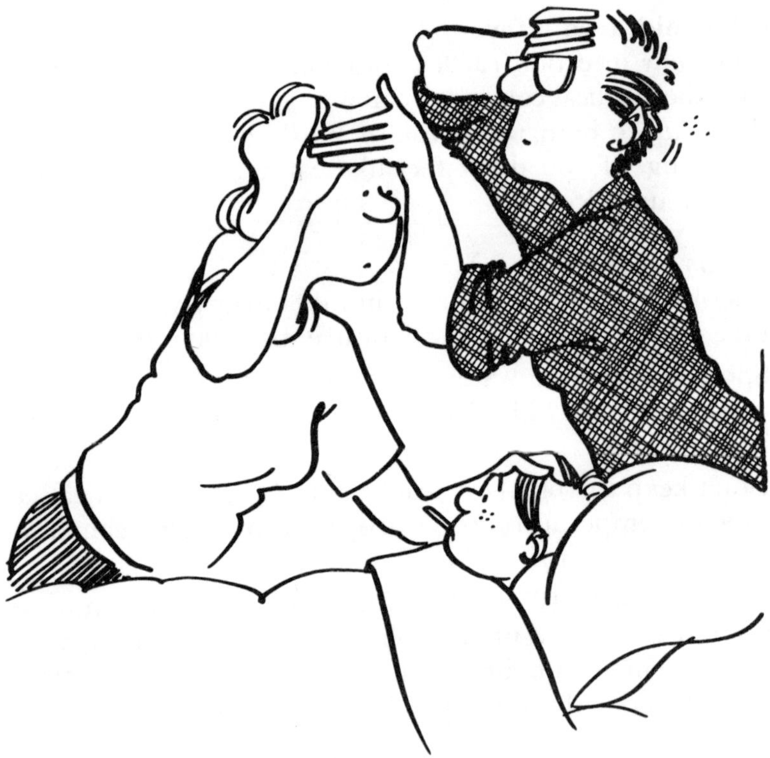

- If the patient is a child, touch your hands and your face to both his forehead and his stomach, then touch a well person.
- But remember: this is only a *rough* gauge of temperature.

Coughing is good for you

- It may make you uncomfortable, but it's nature's way of

clearing the air passages. It's best not to suppress it, but simply to soothe your throat: honey (lots of it) in tea is good.

Be a sourpuss when you have a cough

- Feed your face a pickle, some lemon—anything acidic. Acids help promote the flow of saliva that helps the cough.
- And drink lots of water. It helps liquefy phlegm, making it easier to cough up.

Home remedies for the gargler

- Avoid commercial, chemical-laden gargles and try an herbal tea especially suited for a sore throat. In addition to sage (especially red sage), you could try eucalyptus, fenugreek.
- Or, dissolve two aspirins in a glass of warm water, add ½ teaspoon of baking soda, and stir. Gargle with this four times a day.
- Or, add a pinch of cayenne pepper and a teaspoon of vinegar to horehound tea to which you've added lots of honey.
- Or try ¼ teaspoon of salt in 8 ounces of warm water (about 10 gargles' worth) every two to three hours. Soothing, and the warmth and salt will stimulate circulation, promote healing.
- In any case, gargle gently. You don't have to sound like a motorbike revving up.

Sweet advice for sore throats

- Try a tablespoon of honey and vinegar mixed into your tea. The honey will help soothe the sore throat and relieve coughing, and the vinegar helps break up mucus.

Drag yourself around

- Studies have shown that even a short period of bed rest

can cause dramatic deconditioning. Muscles start to atrophy, bones lose calcium, your blood pressure goes down, and dehydration occurs. So even if you're not feeling your best, don't jump into bed. Stay as active as you can. Of course, if you're really ill, do go to bed. But you'll be back to your old self more quickly if you get up as soon as possible.

Under the Sun

Drugs and sunbathing don't mix

- Certain drugs such as oral contraceptives, tetracycline, some diuretics and tranquilizers make you especially prone to sunburn. Check with your pharmacist.

Makeup's no substitute for sunscreen

- A beauty product must contain at least 3 percent sunscreen to really protect you from the sun. If you're not sure yours does, wear sunscreen under your makeup.

Acne and the sun

- It may feel terrific on your shoulders, but sun doesn't help acne. It actually causes skin to thicken, which could cause more blackheads. Use sunscreen.

Think ahead

- Sunscreen gives you maximum protection if you apply it at least thirty minutes before going out.

Even out the tan

- Changing swimsuit styles in midsummer can leave your

back looking like a patchwork quilt. Don't despair: use sunscreen on the tanned areas and quick-tanning lotion on pale ones. They should balance out in a few days.

Sunburn without sun

- Since ultraviolet light penetrates clouds, bounces off sand and pavement, you should be cautious about exposure. So don't forget to use sunscreen on a cloudy day too.
- Even being "indoors" in a car leaves you vulnerable. Men most often get skin cancer on the left, women on the right, presumably because that's where they sit in the car. So use sunscreen on all exposed skin.

Cover your head in the sun

- As much as thirty percent of body heat is absorbed through the head. White hats reflect heat best.

Stomach Problems

Diet for an upset stomach

- Drink lots of water and flat, non-cola, non-diet soft drinks. They have sugar that stimulates stomach activity.
- Or eat dry foods like unbuttered toast and plain popcorn. They stimulate stomach activity, too.
- It's better to eat small, frequent meals till you feel right again.
- If you're nauseated, try sucking on ice cubes or chips.

Break the antacid habit

- Some antacids contain a large amount of salt and sugar. Read the label if you're on a restricted diet.

- Chronic antacid use inhibits the absorption of iron, magnesium, and phosphorus. It may even break down bones. Use it infrequently.
- If you must take an antacid from time to time, try using baking soda unless you're on a low-sodium diet.
- Or choose a generic or store brand liquid antacid without simethicone. (Liquid works faster than tablets.)

Tips for heartburn sufferers

- Lying down makes the condition worse.
- Drinking milk offers temporary relief, but within the hour the calcium causes the stomach to produce more acid. Avoid it.
- Eating smaller, more frequent meals (five rather than three) may reduce pressure in the stomach.
- Avoid regular and decaffeinated coffee. The caffeine alone increases acid production, and an ingredient in the coffee itself stimulates even more.

Take your ulcer to a Mexican restaurant

- The traditional bland diet is no longer recommended. Only coffee (both regular and decaffeinated) should be avoided, plus any food or spice that particularly irritates you.
- And milk isn't suggested either. Many adults are unable to digest lactose (a milk product) and suffer cramps, gas, bloating or diarrhea.

Withstanding Winter

Dressing for the cold

- If the temperature is 36 degrees, with a windchill factor of −15 degrees, dress for 15-degree weather.
- Wear three layers: the innermost should be absorbent, with a sweatshirt of natural material on top, followed by a windbreaker of cotton (allows sweat to evaporate). Below 20 degrees, add an insulating layer like a turtleneck under the sweatshirt.
- A hat's a must. Most blood vessels contract to save heat in cold weather, but the blood vessels in the head stay open to keep blood going to the brain. That's why you lose 50 percent of body heat through your head.
- For coldest weather, wear long underwear under your pants.
- Mittens are warmer than gloves, since they have less surface area to lose heat. In a pinch, ball up your hands within the mittens.
- Two pairs of thin socks insulate better than one pair of thick ones.
- Wear shoes loose enough so they don't cut off the flow of blood. The blood helps keep feet warm.

Relief for chapped lips

- Try a mix of lemon juice and glycerin.

Cold weather and alcohol don't mix

- Even though it makes you feel warm, alcohol actually causes the blood vessels nearest the surface of the skin to expand, so you lose heat more rapidly. That increases the chance of frostbite.

To keep your mood light

- Winter depression may be associated with increased production of a hormone called melatonin, which your body produces when light is restricted. Remedy: more exposure to ultraviolet rays.
- Try opening windows (glass filters out most ultraviolet rays).
- Go without sunglasses at least part of the time.
- Go on a brief walk at noon when the sun is brightest.

Beware of snow shoveling

- That innocent-looking white stuff can be deadly. Deaths go up after a blizzard, and the vast majority are related to snow shoveling. If you must shovel, rest often, and stop if you overheat, feel your heart pound, or suffer other signs of exertion. Even people in good health can be affected.

Driving in snowy weather

- Carry a colored scarf to tie on the antenna to signal help. You'll be seen in the whiteness.

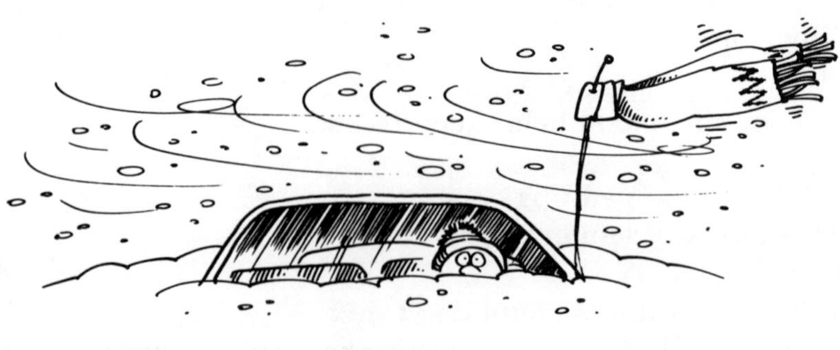

- Keep candles in an empty coffee can for melting snow if you get stuck in a storm, and plastic garbage bags to wrap around you for insulation if you must leave the car.

The Well Worker

It's true: Mondays *are* hazardous to your health

- Now you have a good excuse to take it easy on Mondays: heart attacks are most likely to occur on the first day of the week. This is probably the result of being reexposed to stress on the job, pollutants, and generally increased activity at the beginning of the work week.

For more comfort at your desk

- Put a phone book underneath and prop your feet on it. This will help relieve pressure on your lower back.
- Distribute your weight evenly by sitting on both hips at the same time.
- Put a pillow on the back of your chair, right below your shoulder blades.
- If you must lean over your work, don't hunch your back and shoulders. Instead, bend from your hip sockets.
- Don't twist your torso toward your work; face it head-on.
- Empty your back pockets. Sitting on bulky objects can put pressure on the sciatic nerves in your legs.
- Always keep your feet on the floor or on a book for support.
- Always sit with your knees slightly higher than your hips. Otherwise, your lower back will be stressed.

- Stand up from your desk, stretch, and walk around as often as you can.

Water and work performance

- If your boss complains about your hanging around the water cooler, advise her that lack of water affects work performance more than lack of food. A 4 to 5 percent reduction of body water will result in 20 to 30 percent decline in work performance.

If the chair fits

- You'll work better. People in ill-fitting chairs lose an average of forty minutes of work time daily.
- The test of a good chair: Can you sit with calves and thighs at right angles, and your torso tilted back slightly with support in the small of the back? If not, ask for a new chair.

Quick stress relievers on the job

- Find an empty office and lie down on the carpeted floor. Bend your knees, bring them to your chest, and clasp your hands around them. Gently rock back and forth. Breathe deeply. This will make you feel much better. (Unless you haven't locked the door and your boss stumbles over you!)
- Or, stand in a doorway, pressing one palm against each doorframe. Hold your breath and increase pressure until you feel warmth coming to your neck, face, and head. Hold for as long as you can, then release and inhale deeply. Repeat this three times.

Start fidgeting

- Sitting too long causes swelling in ankles and feet, and sometimes other problems. Do what kids do naturally: squirm, kick your legs, roll your ankles, roll your head around, wring your arms, wrap your arms around your chest.

Pull up a piece of the floor

- Try sitting on the floor for a while each day. It exercises your ball-and-socket hip joint, which never gets worked out if you always sit in a chair.

An out-of-sight exercise

- If you're desk-bound, try slipping off your shoes and rubbing your feet on a rolling pin under the desk. It improves circulation.

Traveling Healthy

Planning a vacation?

- Metabolism is at a peak in July and August, so it's easier to work hard then. The most sensible time for vacationing is periods when you're most likely to feel fatigue: spring and fall.

Going abroad prepared

- If you're taking prescription drugs, pack enough for your trip.
- Carry an extra prescription, written in its *generic name* to make it easier to fill in a foreign country.
- If you combine two kinds of pills in one bottle to save space, label the bottle to remember which is which.
- Take along a supply of your contraceptives. In certain countries they may not be available.
- You might not have broken a pair in the last twenty years, but be sure to take along an extra pair of glasses or contact lenses, as well as your prescription. You don't want to remember the Eiffel Tower or the Taj Mahal as one big blur.

Non-prescription items: a traveler's checklist

- Antacid tablets
- Aspirins
- Sanitary napkins or tampons
- Motion-sickness pills
- Antiseptic spray or lotion
- Adhesive bandages
- Diarrhea medicine
- Eye drops

Avoiding motion sickness

- Children are less likely to get carsick if they can see out the front window of the car.
- Stay near the center of a boat, near the water level, or out on deck. Lie down with eyes open.
- Or try sucking a lemon for seasickness.
- If you feel airsick, look at a point on the distant horizon. This helps decrease the perception of motion.

Avoiding "Montezuma's revenge"

- If you're traveling in a country where food and drink are questionable, particularly avoid salads, and fruit unless you can buy it in its skin.
- Don't drink the water. Remember: this means ordering drinks without ice and brushing teeth with bottled water.

For the long-distance driver

- Researchers have found that drivers who take a break for a hearty meal have better reaction times than those who do not.
- If you want to avoid back problems, be sure you don't have to stretch for the pedals. Adjust your car seat properly, and sit back.

- If you drive a lot, invest in a firm, flat backrest.

A guaranteed lifesaver

- We all know that seat belts save lives, but did you know how much? They reduce the risk of serious injury or death by *50 to 70 percent.* Is that convincing enough for you to buckle up?

For the Flyer

'Ear are a couple of hints for flying

- Try a medication like Ornade, Sudafed Plus, or a nose spray like Afrin or Neo-Synephrine about 1½ hours before descent to relieve those pains in your ears during landing.
- Or cover your ears with plastic cups containing towels or napkins moistened with hot water.

If flying gets you in the stomach

- If your stomach bothers you in planes, it's because decreased atmospheric pressure at high altitudes causes gases to expand. So cut down on gas-producing food, eat slowly, avoid carbonated drinks, and stay away from gum (except during takeoff and landing, when chewing helps unstop your ears).

Fighting jet lag

- Loss of sleep is the main cause of the tiredness, irritability, and mental sluggishness known as jet lag. You may need an over-the-counter sleeping aid to help you snooze on the plane. Then get a good night's sleep on arrival.

• Try to get oriented quickly to local time for sleeping, waking, and eating.

A dietary solution to jet lag

• Change your eating pattern starting three days before your flight: eat normally on the first and third days before departure, but avoid carbohydrates on the second and fourth (departure) days.

• Don't eat or drink alcohol during the flight except a high-protein meal that conforms with the eating schedule of the place to be visited. For example: if flying from New York to Paris on a night flight, ask for breakfast at 2 A.M. New York time, which is 7 A.M. (breakfast time) in Paris.

• On arrival, go through normal schedule, eat a high-protein lunch and high-carbohydrate dinner, then go to bed half an hour earlier than usual.

Legs aching on a long flight?

• Try doing knee raises right in your seat. Pull your knee up toward your chest, then lower it to the floor. Repeat a dozen times with each leg.

Avoiding airsickness

• Fly after dark.

• Get seats away from the engine and toward the center of the plane.

• Ride in a reclining position.

When you fly with kids

• Don't shush your child if he's crying during descent. His ears may be bothering him. Crying's the best thing, since it keeps his ears open.

• If your kid is asleep, wake him before descent and give him a bottle to suck on—or, if an older child, chewing gum.

• No child with a cold or middle-ear infection should fly.

A Good Night's Rest

Best beds

- Sleep experts say that beds that provide the most even pressure distribution are the most beneficial. One university test found that two types were best: an orthopedic 720-coil mattress and box spring, and a standard 10-inch-deep waterbed.
- Avoid "hybrid" beds (those with a central water core topped with foam padding), and soft, 500-coil or less standard beds.
- If you select a foam mattress, get the heaviest one you can find, preferably at least 6 inches thick.

Beddy buys

- Test a mattress by sitting on the edge, then getting up. A good one resumes its shape immediately.
- And lie on the bed, roll to the edge. It should support you, shouldn't tip or sag.
- And check that the mattress doesn't sag, supports your shoulders and hips.

Leg cramps at night

- Try wearing light support hose when you're on your feet, and elevating your legs for about 1 to 1½ hours before bedtime.

How to read in bed

- Don't use pillows to prop yourself up. Instead, use a bed-board that raises the upper half of your body at a 30-degree angle. Put a pillow under your head and a cushion under your knees.

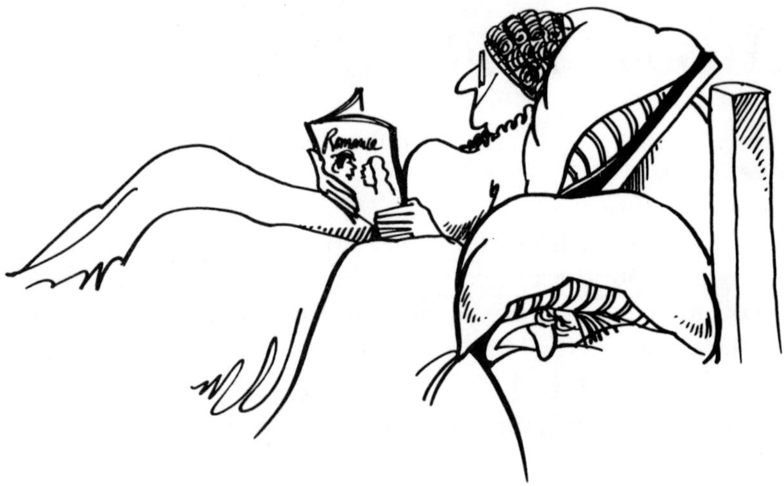

Windows open or windows closed?

- Couples who constantly battle over the issue may reach a truce if they know that you sleep more soundly in a cool room with plenty of ventilation.
- But in *coldest* weather, keep windows closed. Freezing air has too little moisture and brings the humidity (and therefore the comfort level) down.

It's not how much you sleep, it's when you do it

- "Normal" sleep time ranges from six to nine hours, but in adults (and especially in teenagers) what really counts is that it's the *same* hours each night. So try to keep bedtime consistent.

If you're having trouble sleeping

- Go to bed only when you're sleepy.
- Don't associate bed with eating, worrying, reading, watch-

ing TV; think of it only for sleeping—and Casanova's favorite sport.

- If you don't fall asleep in ten minutes, get up, go to another room, lie down again only when you feel sleepy. Repeat if necessary.
- Don't nap during the day.
- Set your alarm for the same time each morning to get your body into a rhythm.

Caffeine keeping you awake?

- Peak stimulation may occur *two to four hours after* you've drunk coffee, causing you to awaken at night or early in the morning. If you can't nod off, break the late-night coffee habit.
- Cut down on caffeine in tea by shortening brewing time. Brewing one minute can result in as little as 9 mg. caffeine, but steep the tea five minutes and your cup will have 30 mg. of caffeine or more.
- Reduce the effect of tannic acid by adding milk to the tea.

Insomnia beater

- It really is true: milk works. That's because it contains a substance that is converted into a brain chemical that works like a sedative. So try a glass of warm milk, or yogurt, or a couple of calcium tablets if you're having trouble dropping off.

Shushing a snorer

- If you're tired of listening to the buzz-saw sounds of your bed partner, don't move to the living room couch. Instead, sew a marble into the back of his pajamas, right between the shoulder blades. Snoring's more likely if someone is lying on his back, and the marble will prod him to turn over.

Easy does it

- Get up in the morning very slooooowly. Jumping out of bed strains your circulatory system, which must readjust to your vertical posture.

If You're on the Weed

Smoking and breathing

- Experts say smoking is a result of needing to breathe deeply. The more shallowly a smoker breathes, the more he's likely to smoke.

Two more reasons to give up smoking

- It ages you quicker. Women who smoke have their menopause one to two years earlier on average than non-smokers.
- Twice as many smokers as non-smokers have peptic ulcers.

There's no such thing as a "safe" smoke

- Harvard and Boston University studies show that risk of heart attack increases with the number of cigarettes but is unrelated to the amount of tar and nicotine the cigarettes contain.

High and dry

- All those "health nuts" who are smoking marijuana ought to know that just one joint can have the same effect on lungs as an entire pack of cigarettes.

Smokers need extra vitamin C

- A pack of cigarettes destroys 500 mg. of vitamin C.

Lip service

- The *British Medical Journal* reports that smokers who left their cigarettes hanging from their lips had a much greater rate of chronic bronchitis than those who removed it from their mouths between puffs.

Smoking and blood pressure

- Smoking only one cigarette increases the level of adrenaline in the blood by 25 percent, which constricts blood vessels and raises blood pressure. Don't kid yourself that smoking "only a little" is okay.

It *does* pay to quit

- Your body can heal when you stop smoking. In fact, smokers who had the worst lung impairment showed the greatest improvement on all tests after they stopped. Symptoms such as coughing, wheezing, and shortness of breath disappeared almost completely. So don't say "it's too late" to quit.

Whatever Ails You

Acne

- It might comfort your teenager to know that 86 percent of American kids seventeen and younger have some form of acne.

Chocolate's okay—but lay off the clams

- Doctors now say that chocolate doesn't aggravate acne. Foods that do include nuts, foods containing iodine (shrimp, lobster, clams), and seaweed and kelp (health food items). Fast food may also cause acne, *possibly* because of the iodine-containing cleansers that sterilize the machines.

Allergies

- About one in every ten people gets an allergic reaction to nickel, which is used in many watches, earrings, rings, and bracelets. If your skin's been irritated, your jewelry may be the culprit.
- All the over-the-counter medicine contains approximately the same ingredients, so choose the cheapest one.
- If antihistamines make you drowsy, choose chlorpheniramine instead.
- Clean out the air conditioner before the season starts. Allergy-causing substances may have accumulated over winter.

Tax deductible allergy

- It might ease your suffering (or at least your pocketbook) a bit to know that the cost of purchasing and/or running an air conditioner is a tax deduction if you have an allergy. Check with the I.R.S. about filing a claim.

Back problems

- Doctors often recommend rocking chairs for people with chronic back problems who have to sit for long periods.
- Try keeping a leg up. The footrail in pubs was designed to do this for you. At home, get the same effect by putting your foot on a low stool or chair.

Broken bones

- A bit of good news: the new plastic casts with foam inner sleeves can be removed for bathing or showering, permit certain exercises that reduce swelling and speed healing. So if you have the bad luck to break a bone, at least you'll know the cast may be easier to wear and you may heal quicker than in the past.

Cellulite

- Since cellulite is just fat, no matter what you've heard, you *can* do something about it: diet and exercise.
- Diet to your appropriate weight, then get on a schedule of walking for an hour five times a week. Buttocks and thigh muscles are used in a pulling motion that greatly helps firm up these areas.

Eyeache

- Relieve an aching eye by pressing the inside corner of the *other* eye.

Hiccups

- Swallow a teaspoonful of dry granulated sugar and they'll go away.
- Or try saturating a lemon wedge in Angostura bitters and eating the entire wedge (but not the rind).

Minor discomforts

- A sustained pinch of the area between nose and upper lip has been reported to relieve such problems as leg cramp, hiccups, lower back spasms, and other ailments.

Premenstrual syndrome (PMS)

- If you reduce the amount of salt you eat for the week before you expect your period, you may reduce bloating.
- Try hot baths, hot compresses, and massage for cramps.
- Take aspirin (or one of the aspirin substitutes). But you don't need all the other stuff that's mixed into the expensive menstrual cramp remedies.
- Try rubbing in the middle of the back about an inch to the right of your spine. Pain from cramps should subside within thirty seconds and disappear within minutes. It will not return for three to six hours.

Skin injury

- Try rubbing the sap from a piece of an aloe vera plant on a minor skin injury such as a burn or cut.

Urinary tract infection

- Cranberry juice is an aid in fighting urinary tract infection and may even help prevent it. Most bacteria can't live in an acidic environment, which the cranberry juice helps create.

Vocal cord strain

- If your vocal cords are tired from too much talking, try yawning, then sighing. (If you're *really* talking too much, you may notice others around you doing the same thing.)

Warts

- In one study, daily applications of vitamin A-enriched cod-liver oil cleared up the warts of most of the patients.

Coping with the Environment

The city vs. the country

- Where are you less likely to suffer mental illness? Surprisingly, it's more common with rural than city dwellers. Possible reasons include greater isolation and more economic hardship in rural areas.

The industrial-strength vitamin

- Vitamin A helps protect the lining of the lungs. People who live in large industrial cities should be sure to get the recommended daily amount of this nutrient through eating foods rich in it, such as yellow and dark green vegetables, or by taking vitamin supplements.

The moon and illness

- Certain physical ailments seem to be linked with the moon. Ulcers seem more likely to bleed, and heart attacks are more likely during the full moon. Possible cause: effect of the moon on the earth's magnetic field.

Warning to craftspeople

- Potters may be exposing themselves to asbestos, and silk-screen artists to dangers from ink and solvents. Find out more about your materials in the *Health Hazards Manual for Artists.* Send $3.50 plus $1.00 for postage to: Art Hazards Information Center, 5 Beekman Street, New York, NY 10038

Relief from poison ivy

- Pour two cups of milk into a quart container, then fill it up by adding ice cubes plus two tablespoons of salt. Apply to infected area with a cloth for twenty minutes, three or four times daily. This works for bug bites and sunburn, too.
- Or see if you can buy some plantain leaves at your local nursery. Crush them and apply to the affected area, repeating if necessary. Your itch should stop.

Don't read the label

- Studying over 1,000 common household products, the New York City Poison Control Project found that over 85 percent gave wrong, incomplete, or dangerous instructions. If you suspect poisoning, call your local poison-control center. (Be sure you have its number near the phone.)
- And always have ipecac on hand.

Love and Laughter

Garlic or a good-night kiss

- If you want to mix garlic and romance, mix your raw garlic in salad. Allicin (the chemical that causes its strong odor) will be diluted by the chlorophyll and fiber in the greens.

Pucker up for health and profit

- Men who kiss their wives before leaving for work are healthier, live longer, and earn more money, a study shows. (It helps them start the day with a positive attitude.)

If he hasn't popped the question, tell him this

- Married men are nearly eight times less likely than bachelors to have severe emotional problems or breakdowns.

I'm okay if you're okay, dear

- A man's satisfaction in old age appears to depend more on his wife's emotional stability and health than on his own.

Love a pet

- Pet owners recover from sicknesses (including heart attacks) better than non-pet owners. Any kind of pet counts, even a gerbil.

Comedy and romance

- If you're in the mood for romance, treat your guy or gal to a funny movie. After being stimulated by laughter, people are more responsive to other stimuli—including the opposite sex.

Laughter *is* the best medicine

- A hearty laugh gives a workout to your stomach and chest muscles, heart and lungs. And though your blood pressure and adrenaline go up during laughter, they drop right down to normal or below afterward, releasing stress.

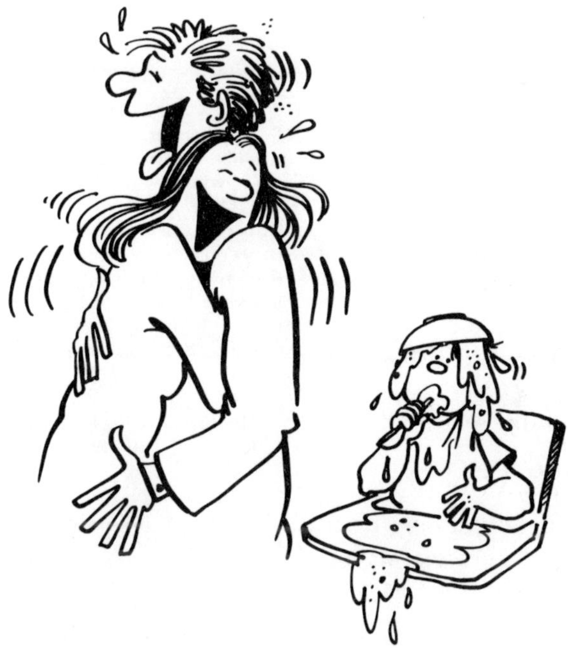

Index

Also available from Doubleday

Mary Ellen Family Books™

Mary Ellen Family Books

Mary Ellen Family Books

BABY'S FIRST HELPINGS

Superhealthy Meals for Superhealthy Kids

Chris Casson Madden

ISBN: 0-385-19143-X comb-bound paperback $5.95

TAKING CARE OF MOMMY

Everything Your Doctor Wouldn't, Your Mother Couldn't, and Your Best Friend Didn't Tell You About Becoming a Mommy

Susan G. Gross and Paula S. Linden, R.D.

ISBN: 0-385-19144-8 paperback $7.95

THE MILLION DOLLAR CONTEST COOKBOOK

Jean Sanderson

ISBN: 0-385-19145-6 comb-bound paperback $6.95

GREAT BEGINNINGS, GREAT ENDINGS

Make Ahead Hors d'oeuvres and Desserts

Carol Sakstrup and Jane Charboneau

ISBN: 0-385-19146-4 comb-bound paperback $3.95

GIFT OF FRIENDSHIP COUPONS

Patti Brietman and Nanc Gordon

ISBN: 0-385-19218-5 paperback $3.95

---

500 HINTS FOR KIDS

Randy Harleson and Eileen Cavanaugh

ISBN: 0-385-19217-7 paperback $5.95

RUMMAGE, TAG & GARAGE SALES

For Profit & Fun!

Irma and R.A. Pohl

ISBN: 0-385-19505-2 paperback $4.95

OUTSMART THE SAT'S

Kathryn Kendall

ISBN: 0-385-19506-0 paperback $8.95
